the gut stuff

First published in the United Kingdom in
2024 by Pavilion
An imprint of HarperCollinsPublishers Ltd
1 London Bridge,
London, SE1 9GF

www.harpercollins.co.uk

HarperCollinsPublishers
Macken House
39/40 Mayor Street Upper
Dublin 1
D01 C9W8
Ireland

10 9 8 7 6 5 4 3 2

First published in Great Britain by Pavilion
An imprint of HarperCollinsPublishers 2024

ISBN 978-0-00-862151-3

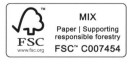

This book contains FSC™ certified paper
and other controlled sources to ensure
responsible forest management.

For more information visit:
www.harpercollins.co.uk/green

Publishing Director: Stephanie Milner
Commissioning Editor: Kiron Gill
Editorial Assistant: Shamar Gunning
Design Director: Laura Russell
Design Assistant: Lily Wilson
Layout Designer: James Boast
Senior Production Controller: Grace O'Byrne
Infographics design: Scarlett Chetwin,
Harry Lee and Myron Darlington at Revolt
Logos and branding: James Knowles Ritchie

Photography credits:
page 8 Josh Exell
page 35 Emma Croman
page 48 Joe Pollard

Printed in Malaysia

the gut stuff

your ultimate guide to a happy and healthy gut

Alana & Lisa Macfarlane

PAVILION

what's inside?

– other than your gut ;)

foreword

As Director of the Department of Twin Research at King's College London I have come across many thousands of twins over the years. None are like the Mac twins! Alana and Lisa have an amazing infectious enthusiasm, intelligence and passion for research, and disseminating that science to the public. They quickly became my go-to twin guinea pigs to road-test new research projects.

I met them around 10 years ago when they answered my call to participate on an epigenetic research project where I was looking at why identical twins could often look identical but be quite different in many ways. They ended up being a great case study in my book, *Identically Different*, with their different personalities and gut problems. Lisa and Alana then eagerly volunteered for more studies and went on to be the very first participants in a pilot study for our novel research project into the gut microbiome and nutrition. This study involved having all kinds of biopsies, plenty of poo samples and eating several weeks of junk food. Luckily they were performing at the Edinburgh festival where this was readily available. They survived this ordeal followed by four weeks of healthy vegetarian high-fibre food. Their results showed us that we could alter the gut microbes with diet and allowed us to start a bigger study with hundreds more twins, and open up the whole field of research.

The research evolved into the world's largest personalised nutrition study with the help of a company called ZOE – titled the PREDICT program. The twins were, once again, the first guinea pigs and had to say how they reacted differently to the identical foods, blue muffins, (and prosecco). Lisa and Alana made the point brilliantly of how unique all of us are. They both were fascinated by the science of the trillions of microbes living in our gut that are essential to our immunity and overall health, as well as how looking after them through a diverse and varied diet could help prevent many modern health conditions. As identical twins they were used to sharing all their genes, but suddenly they had something that was unique to only them – the microbes in their gut. Throughout their participation in the research, they never stopped asking ever tougher and more intelligent questions about the science of the microbiome and, most importantly, they showed a unique talent not just for processing complicated scientific concepts but for translating them to a non-scientific audience in a fun and highly informative manner.

I was not surprised when they went on to found the incredibly successful The Gut Stuff, a platform to empower gut health for everyone.

This book is the next step in their efforts to make microbes, the science of gut health and nutrition available for everyone and show that science does not have to be boring. Through their ability to attract and talk to the best experts in the field they have managed to summarise a wealth of scientific knowledge and different viewpoints to educate a young audience on what they need to do to maintain and enhance their health. I was asked on a nutrition panel recently – what single factor is the most important in changing nutrition? I replied, 'educating everybody, even at school'. As my own books, *The Diet Myth* and *Spoon-Fed* underline, there is a real need for better nutritional health that demystifies food and nutrition. Alana and Lisa's book deserves top place in the list of books every young and not-so-young person should read, because as they themselves say, "Gut health is serious shit". Enjoy.

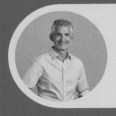

Tim Spector
Professor of Genetic Epidemiology, King's College London
Author of *Food for Life* (2022), *Spoon-Fed* (2020) and *The Diet Myth* (2016).

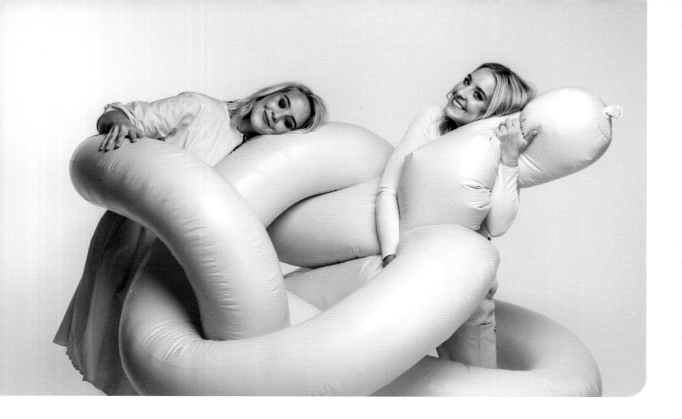

introduction

Let's face it, talking about the gut ain't sexy. Just googling 'gut' brings up a rather disturbing mosaic of beer bellies, intestinal diagrams and, the main reason for our misconceptions – perfectly manicured hands, cupping toned, soft stomachs. It's no wonder we're all so confused.

So many of us have digestive issues at any given time, but we'd rather talk about ANYTHING other than our gurgling midriff and toilet dashing. So from this sentence on is where that STOPS. You are now entering an open 'poo chat' forum and you wanna know why? Because it's important, really important. Hippocrates saw it many moons ago when he said:

 "all disease begins in the gut"

For some reason we've chosen to bury that knowledge. So, get your little archaeological spades and hats out, as we're about to discover what Hippocrates was on about, for the good of our health.

Look, nutrition is COMPLEX. Even the experts say so and, trust us, we were not experts. We had done every fad diet under the sun, including the cabbage soup diet in 2005 (remember that?), and, we also grew up in Scotland eating deep-fried pizza and fries, plus most of Edinburgh's supply of yum-yums. We only knew what kale was because we used to feed it to the guinea pig on his birthday. That all flip-reversed when we volunteered to be part of the TwinsUK research at King's College London.

Being identical twins, we have a passion (teetering on obsession) for finding out what's different about us and to do this we looked inside ourselves, as there wasn't much different on the outside. Twins are a great constant for medical research, and we became the 'chief guinea pigs' for the British Gut Project. We discovered that despite having 100% of the same DNA, our guts share only 30–40% of the same microbiota, which could explain why our bodies behave so differently. And so our 'gut journey' began and now yours will too.

Between 2015 and 2020, Google searches for gut health increased by over 400%. Far from being a flying fad, the microbiome market is skyrocketing, so why is everyone still so bloomin' confused? And more importantly why are 'gut health' conversations only happening in health food stores and hot yoga queues? Why hasn't the message reached the wider population, and especially the people who suffer the most?

With the science being pretty new (and at times conflicting) it makes for a difficult world to navigate, so KNOWLEDGE is POWER. Fortunately, we've grown an expert team of scientists, dietitians, nutritionists, and doctors to keep us all on the right side of the tracks – many of whom you'll meet in these pages. We were expecting futuristic toilets seats that scan our poos, a pill filled with all our digestive hopes and dreams, and maybe even a miracle cure. But what did they tell us? Simple stuff, like eat more fibre, cut down on ultra-processed foods, look at how you're sleeping and managing your stress levels. Drink water, for goodness' sake! Everything our granny used to tell us!

Gut health is brilliantly complex – because it's so important – but how we speak about it doesn't have to be. Everyone deserves to know their gut – they've got it for life, after all.

Whether you're here because you're struggling with digestive issues, you've heard lots of chatter about 'the gut' recently and want to know what all the fuss is about or just for the polyphenLOLs (you'll get that joke soon), welcome to the Gut Gang.

Once you have learnt the science and how to 'live that gut life' we'll be welcoming you to The Gut Stuff dinner table, and you CAN sit with us. We're laying out the table of misconceptions, pouring a smooth glass of 'why' and serving a plentiful helping of 'how'.

Think of this as snacking at the back of a biology lesson; dip in and out, try and read the juicy bits and make sure you pass along your favourite parts to your classmates. We peer into the wonderful world of food through the magnificent lens of gut health, but we'd like you to add on 'your health' at the end of the telescope – this is your toolkit.

We were also both kinda fed up of gut-friendly recipes that needed ingredients we couldn't find, so we've made sure there is absolutely something in here for everyone – if Alana can do it, anyone can! Lisa, on the other hand, really enjoys cooking and is the hostess with the mostest at dinner parties – but whichever camp you fall into, or somewhere in between, we hope you get a lot of use out of this book, and that it gets suitably marked with stains and your own little notes throughout.

Lisa and Alana x

Disclaimer: This book isn't going to make you a gourmet chef with impeccable culinary prowess. It isn't going to have you scouring the supermarkets for the newest, most unusual ingredients to impress your dinner guests, nor is it going to transform your plates into the envy of the Instagram #foodie. It goes way deeper than that – to explore what is there inside you... literally.

why now?

We've always had guts – so why are we all just talking about the gut now?

There's stuff we've known for a pretty long time, for example, that the gut is pretty clever and acts like our second brain, even communicating how we feel. (The gut and brain actually work much more closely together than we thought – more on this later.) Aside from just how fascinating the gut is, with so many people encountering digestive issues, there's a huge demand to know more. Even if you don't have digestive problems, looking after your gut is still as important as looking after your heart and all your other bits and bobs. Here's a rundown of some of the main reasons we're all talking about our guts.

Looking back to 1990 there were approximately twenty-four studies on the microbiota published that year; fast forward to 2019–2020 and there were over 9,000 studies in just one year, bringing it to a total of over 40,000 in thirty years – that's a lot of research. NOTE: this includes all microbiota, ranging from the gut to the skin. Despite all this research, we only know a fraction of what our gut does and how powerful it really is.

1. First up, we're learning more about the microbiota (jump to page 16) and what our gut bugs and travelling bugs do for and against us. Many bacteria don't like to be exposed to air, so when scientists were trying to study them out of the body, they died – so we had limited knowledge about them. Now we have the technology to study the DNA of these little guys instead of attempting to grow them in labs, which is why we are making so many advances in getting to know them better.

2. Digestive issues are on the rise; 86% of all British adults have suffered some form of gastrointestinal (GI) problem or ailment in the last year, encountering symptoms ranging from bloating and excessive wind to crippling pain and chronic disease.

3. In the Western world, we've forgotten about our gut microbes, along with our Walkmans and VCRs and we have increased our consumption of ultra-processed foods bursting with additives and emulsifiers, which aren't great for our microbes.

4. Despite the availability and variety of unprocessed food being greater than ever, the majority of us aren't getting enough fibre (see page 100 for more), which has a huge impact on our gut microbes.

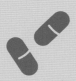

5. While antibiotics have saved many lives, used incorrectly or without the right support, they can act like a nuclear bomb on our gut microbes, affecting the balance between the beneficial and less helpful microbes and even wiping out entire species altogether.

6. We've also created a very sterile environment with our hand rubs and bleaches (rightly so at times), but in the process we've killed off some good microbes we actually need.

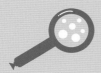

7. Our sterile environment coupled with more sedentary lifestyles and spending too much time in our homes may be damaging our health.

Now that we know the *why*, it's time to go back to school and learn the *what* before we get onto the *how* (this is like a game of Cluedo!).

chapter 1

the
science

back to school

We say "gut" – you say "what" – "gut" – "what"... stay with us...

'Gut health' is a vague term and isn't as clear cut as other areas of health (like heart health) and there is still so much we are discovering...

When we talk about gut health, we are referring to the health of two different things:

1. The gastrointestinal tract
(aka your gut – which is nearly five metres long!)

2. Gut microbiota
(we will call them gut microbes throughout)

These two things work in harmony with the rest of your body and have a profound impact on health.

Since this isn't actually school and we can do what the hell we like, we thought we'd mash up a biology and music class seeing as our gut is a wonderful orchestra, and we don't just mean the trumpet at the end. The surface area of our digestive system is forty times larger than our skin and there are several organs involved (and not the church kind). That's a lot of orchestra seats and stands, with Mother Nature as the best conductor of all. There will be a lot of music references across these pages, the by-product of two DJ's writing a book about science.

what is the gut?

Cells lining your gut secrete enzymes and juices into the lumen (the hollow bit) and hormones into the blood.

starts here

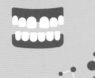

Pharynx
Pushes food into your oesophagus (food pipe).

Oesophagus
Quick ride straight to your stomach.

Liver
Produces bile to help you digest fats (and has many more other functions – it's a clever beast).

Gallbladder
Like your liver's sidekick, it stores bile ready for when it's needed.

Stomach
Strong muscles mix up your food with stomach acid (hydrochloric acid) and enzymes to both mechanically and chemically break down your food into something called chyme (pronounced *kaim*).

Small intestine
Here is where a lot of enzymes get to work digesting your food further and where the majority of nutrients are absorbed.

Pancreas
Produces and releases pancreatic juice, including enzymes, which neutralize chyme and support the breakdown of carbohydrates, proteins and fats.

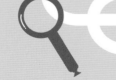

Your gastrointestinal tract (or GI tract)
This is actually a flexible hollow tube made up of lots of layers, including a mucosa, which is home to some interesting species of bacteria. Your mucosa is a physical barrier that separates you from your microbes, it works hard to defend you, can change the make-up of microbes in your gut and some bacteria even feast on it!

Large intestine
If food isn't digested in the small intestine, it passes into your large intestine for further digestion and this is where the majority of your gut microbes live.

Rectum

ends here

"What's my gut? Just my stomach yeah?"

Your stomach isn't actually your gut but one player in tune with other organs, including your liver, gallbladder and pancreas, working in harmony to support your gut. Yes, it can sound more like death metal than Bach at times, but all the players are there with their parts ready and willing it to work.

We shall call this aria, 'To eat: the long journey out'.

Our mouth is the perfect introduction to the show, with a plodding duet of your teeth and saliva working together to break down your food both physically (teeth) and chemically (by clever enzymes contained in your saliva). Their tunes dance round each other with the same aim: to get the food as small as possible to make it easier for the next key players to read the sheet music. But too many of us don't let the tunes play for long enough – cue not chewing – making it hard for the next players to continue playing.

side note ♪♫

If you thought your tongue was just for tasting, you've very much underestimated it – there are actually immune cells at the back of our tongue that are 'on guard' ready to protect us. More on them later...

The oesophagus is like a didgeridoo with a sphincter (valve) at the top and bottom that moves food from the back of your throat to your stomach. This is not to be confused with your windpipe (the clarinet next door). You'll know if these two have ever been confused *spluttering cough*. The sphincter at the top stops air going in and the sphincter at the bottom allows food to enter the stomach but prevents the acidic contents of your stomach going up.

And now for the stomach, the big clever bagpipe, which acts as an expensive mixer to churn our food into chyme (another musical reference nearly hit, but not quite).

side note ♪♫

Our stomach is a lot higher up than we think (see page 17), so often when people complain of stomach ache, it's not actually stomach ache, it's probably something a lot further down the line.

Firstly, the stomach separates solids from liquids. The liquids get a VIP fast track onto the next phase, but the solids have to be mixed up in the queue a little longer.

myth bust

"It's bad if our stomach is really acidic."

WRONG. Our stomach needs to have a low pH (acidic) to break down our food; the enzymes really like an acid party up in there and they need it to get rid of the unwanted 'microbes' that weren't invited.

And so, to the small intestine where the song starts to gain momentum, as it's got a lot of pals to help the process. Nutrients are absorbed here by the villi, which we think look like sea anemones, and the food is here for 2–6 hours (it's a long tune!).

side note ♪♫

The small intestine is lined with tiny finger-like structures called villi. The inner wall of villi is only one cell thick, so it's a sensitive Sally, and it's pretty easy for substances to pass in and out of it (so not a soundproof music hall). Some foods and medications, excessive alcohol and stress may make Sally feel a bit out of sorts and she might occasionally let substances – like food particles and toxins produced by bacteria – into the bloodstream that she shouldn't.

In comes the liver, like a big important double bass (arguably the most important organ, which is why it deserves its own bullet points). The liver tends to command a lot of attention (and rightly so) because it does so many things, the key ones being:

- Produces bile acids that 'skoosh' in via the gallbladder, which is a trusty sidekick that stores all the bile acids (not to be confused with hangover sickness) when the time is right – like a steady cello perhaps?

- Filters blood coming from the small intestine, in doing so it:

  - 'polices' what's in the blood, such as toxins or medications, which it then has a good sort through and either turns them into something less harmful or metabolizes them.

  - converts food to fuel to give us energy (even our gut needs energy to work).

  - stores vitamins, minerals, fats and sugar for later use.

- Produces hormones to help regulate lots of different functions around our body.

To round off the string section is the pancreas, which secretes enzymes and hormones that play a part in controlling blood sugar and sodium bicarbonate to change the pH of chyme that enters your small intestine and other things.

Hold up! Chyme? Whaaat?!

What is it? A cocktail of stomach acid, digestive enzymes, partially digested food and water.
What does it do? Chyme allows for further digestion by enzymes and carries food and enzymes to the small intestine.

Into the plodding adagio we move, as all the unabsorbed bits of food make their way into the large intestine (for around 12–30 hours – hope everyone brought snacks to this show). Here is where most of our gut microbes live (more on this after the show) and they LOVE everything that our human enzymes can't break down, like fibre.

side note ♪♫

We forgot about the appendix. (Most people do.) It's got a reputation for being the spare part, like the cow bell. It sits just below the junction between the small and large intestine and is seemingly completely bypassed. However, just like the cow bell in the Christmas nativity (nothing else can signify donkey steps quite like a cow bell), it isn't just there for show. Some experts believe the appendix is like a big storage container for all the most helpful bacteria ready for when we need them most, like when we have diarrhoea.

AND SO FOR THE BIG CRESCENDO, aka getting it out the other end. This is our last chance to absorb any water. The music (hopefully the poo) swells as our intestinal muscles push along your poo to sit in the waiting room (your rectum)… the music stops dramatically… as our external sphincter closes, ready for the opportune time to introduce the trumpet and complete the song.

The audience are in POO-sitition (pages 75–77 for how to do this optimally), the brain signals it's time for the eagle to land and the final trumpet sings the final notes – *DADADADAAAAAAAA!*

A round of applause, not dissimilar to the sound of a flush, and the audience are on their feet (washing their hands). *What a show!*

And if that wasn't enough, there's also a whole other neighbouring orchestra waiting in the wings to help out too… enter THE MICROBIOME.

microbiome 101

To rephrase Ellie Goulding, 'When I'm with ME, I'm standing with an army.'

We are not all human. (Don't worry, you've not dipped into a sci-fi novel in which fourteen-fingered extraterrestrials escape from your intestines to conquer the world as we know it.) No, we have well over a million little critters like bacteria, viruses, fungi and other organisms just chillin' in and around our body, mostly in our large intestine, also known as our gut microbiome. It's a bit like a tropical jungle with loads of different species living and working in harmony. Now, if you'd told us this a couple of years ago, we would've wanted to chuck them right off our turf and out onto the street without an eviction notice. However, it turns out we need them.

Despite our microbes being scattered around the body, scientists are starting to treat them as an organ within their own right. Welcome to the stage little bugs, your time has come to shine *in the style of Simon and Garfunkel*. Scientists are discovering that not only do our microbes outnumber our genes, but they are potentially just as influential. If this were *Game of Thrones*, they would be an army we definitely want to have on board. They are devoted to us from birth and maybe even before (thanks Mum) – even if in the Western world we've unknowingly been doing all we can to deplete them (treason!). But more on that later. All these microbes are exceptionally clever and help to control your blood sugar, produce vitamins, manage cholesterol and hormonal balance, prevent you from getting infections, control the calories that you absorb and store, communicate with your nervous system and brain, and influence your bone strength, alongside hundreds of other functions!

Similar to the sage advice Aibileen gives Mae Mobley in one of our favourite film quotes from *The Help*, our microbes are kind, smart and important.

Kind

Microbes protect us. They know the difference between harmful party crashers like pathogens and harmless holiday-makers just fancying a journey through your intestines.

Smart

Microbes are much more agile than our human cells. They can reshape and cultivate according to their environment – absolute ninjas. They can actually swap genes and bits of DNA amongst themselves, like a tiny miniature microbe stock exchange.

Important

Microbes affect pretty much everything: including our ability to break down food, absorb nutrients, make vitamins, regulate appetite and produce feel-good hormones. They can even inhibit the production of hormones that make us feel happy (blows our minds every time!).

Your gut microbiota may also play an important role in the development of Alzheimer's and Parkinson's disease, attention deficit hyperactivity disorder (ADHD), autism, diabetes, obesity, polycystic ovary syndrome (PCOS) and autoimmune conditions and it can also influence your cardiovascular health. Most of the research points towards gut-microbiota-driven inflammation being key in the development of many of these conditions, but we are really just on the precipice of discovering exactly how different species of bacteria can help decrease or increase the risk of developing such illnesses.

The robustness of this community of microbes can make a huge, huge difference to our health, and the most fantastic news is – we can change it ourselves. Goodness knows we need to...

In the Western world we've neglected our clever microbes by: consuming processed foods bursting with additives and emulsifiers; living fast-paced, stressful lives; dedicating our brains to devices late at night, impacting our sleep; and probably not getting as much movement as we should. All of which, combined, wreak havoc on our garden of microbes, resulting in it looking more like a vegetable patch that's lost its scarecrow than a beautiful, colourful lawn.

We can't say for definite what a healthy microbiome should look like, but we do know microbial diversity is associated with health. So, we need to start taking care of our microbial friends and making new ones. It doesn't have to be drastic, break the bank or involve weird cleanses (visit our Bullsh*t Bin for more, pages 90–92). There are some really simple things you can do to meet new bacterial recruits and help the ones you already have flourish. We've gut you covered with some gut-loving tips and tricks to pick up (see pages 98–103).

Now, we know what you're thinking, "How on earth am I going to employ an army without a job description or any idea what these microbes do?!"

Role: Epithelium protector/bad ass

Length of contract: A lifetime

Payment: Health

Description:

The mucus-producing intestinal epithelium lines our digestive tract and is just one cell thick. It is fundamental for immune function and forms the first line of defence, separating your self from your non-self. It's like a skin, which when stretched out would cover a tennis court, and our gut microbes are absolutely critical to its health. If the epithelium is not looked after properly, it can become papery and penetrable, like a colander. Substances can get through it to have a swim in our bloodstream, including endotoxins (that's toxic substances bound to bacteria to you and me), proteins and other food components. This can cause an emergency response from our immune system – *sound the alarm* – 'WE HAVE INTRUDERS!' And so, inflammation, part of your body's immune response, is triggered. Don't get us wrong, inflammation at the right time and place is a perfectly normal response, but like the guy at the bar who just won't leave, it can cause problems further down the line if it lingers on too long (becoming chronic). Chronic inflammation is linked to metabolic disorders such as diabetes, rheumatoid arthritis, heart disease, gastrointestinal disorders, poor mental health and many more. So, it is no laughing matter, and your intestinal epithelium plays a very important role.

Your intestinal epithelium cells get replaced every 4–5 days! So, changes can be made really quickly. High staff turnover, eh? HR nightmare!

Some bacteria can directly enhance the epithelium's function, namely *Lactobacillus plantarum* (aka a tongue twister), which can be found in fermented vegetables. So, whoever receives this role must be in possession of high quantities of sauerkraut.

Now, back to that mucus lining. What's this got to do with bacteria? *Akkermansia muciniphila* (another catchy name) is a bacteria with health-promoting benefits, which loves a bit of fasting, lives off your mucus lining and is associated with people who have a lower body mass index (BMI). If your mucus layer is damaged, say by too much alcohol (oops), it can reduce the amount of *Akkermansia* kicking about. See where we are going with this? Bacteria influences almost everything. Stress, too much alcohol and processed food can all influence your delicate gut lining, so tune in and take control to help keep self away from non-self. Apply within.

gut microbiome 101

Your gut microbiome is a term used to describe the microorganisms present in your gut (mostly your large intestine). Here are just a few of the things they do for you:

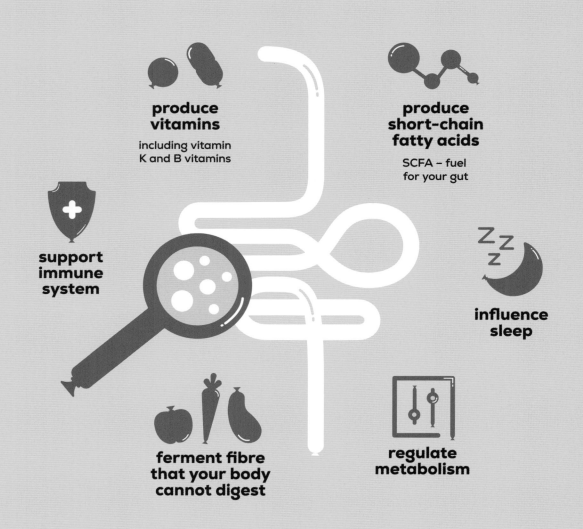

produce vitamins

including vitamin K and B vitamins

produce short-chain fatty acids

SCFA – fuel for your gut

support immune system

influence sleep

ferment fibre that your body cannot digest

regulate metabolism

Our microbes perform a list of jobs long enough to overload even the most prolific job centre, but it's an army we can build and cultivate ourselves. The research is still very, very new and, in some cases, conflicting. But at some point in the future, alongside self-driving cars, jars that open with ease and a phone battery invented by the Duracell bunny, the research will be so advanced and healthcare so personalized that we'll know exactly what bacteria we need and have a lovely little probiotic and prebiotic made just for us to chug down with our morning coffee. Until then, there are simple changes (and wonderful additions) that we'll introduce you to in this book, while the scientists are beavering away.

OK, so we know we have these other friends. We know where they live. We know where they work. But what makes them tick and what are they affected by?

what influences your gut microbes?

– quite a lot as it turns out!

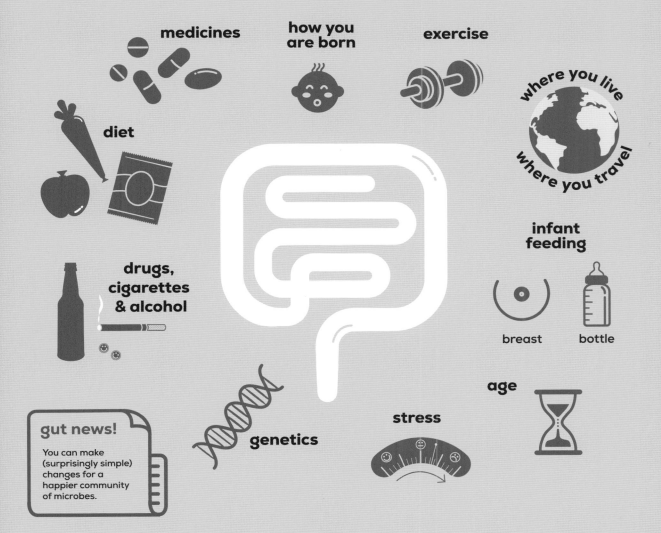

medicines

how you are born

exercise

diet

where you live where you travel

drugs, cigarettes & alcohol

infant feeding

breast   bottle

age

gut news!

You can make (surprisingly simple) changes for a happier community of microbes.

genetics

stress

The final lesson for the day to give us all a bit of context is...

modern studies and politics

Don't worry, this isn't a test on British voting systems or the welfare state, but class and politics have been linked with nutrition and health since the beginning of time, and it's the reason we started our business. This comes down to access to information, private healthcare, accessibility of language and sources and, of course, cash. Most of us just see health as 'not being ill' and 'well-being' as a middle-class world of luxury occupied by green smoothies and gong baths. In fact, it is VITAL we start to think of them together if we want to turn our focus to prevention rather than cure and help take the strain off our healthcare system.

Dr Chris George is an NHS doctor, and all his advice on lifestyle is based on scientific research, evidence, and his clinical experience as a doctor. He's also director of the British Society of Lifestyle Medicine, so there's no better person to teach this part of the lesson...

"The World Health Organization (WHO) reported that 71% of deaths worldwide are due to chronic lifestyle-related conditions termed 'non-communicable diseases', including illnesses such as cancer, stroke and heart disease. Chronic conditions are actually the largest cause of death and disability, but these chronic conditions are largely preventable through the modification of lifestyle factors such as diet and exercise. Diet and nutrition are important factors in maintaining good health. Despite increased awareness that poor diet is associated

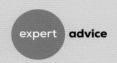

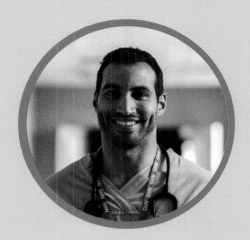

Dr Chris George

with negative health outcomes, food choice remains an extremely complex subject. Within our healthcare system, socioeconomic status (SES) and education appear to be the largest determining factors when it comes to nutrition. There are numerous studies that show people's diet can be related to their SES. This means that the consumption of an unhealthy diet, classically one low in fruit and vegetables, is associated with people from poorer backgrounds. Less nutritious, energy-dense foods are typically cheaper sources of calories, whereas a higher quality diet tends to cost more. People who shop at low-priced supermarkets have been shown to have lower quality diets and higher BMIs. Interestingly, this cannot be put down to cost alone, as people from higher educated households shopping within the same supermarket have been shown to make healthier food selections.

What we're seeing in clinical practice is a rise in most gastrointestinal (GI) disorders, including functional GI disorders, alcohol-related disease and rising obesity levels. Functional GI disorders, such as irritable bowel syndrome (IBS), are incredibly common and sufferers are often not seeking the help that they need from their doctor. This means that they are living with debilitating disorders, which are having a huge impact on their work and home lives. In addition, access to specialist nutritional advice is often too expensive for many patients living with chronic digestive diseases, which can exacerbate healthcare inequalities. Furthermore, with huge amounts of misinformation and health myths on social media, it's hard to find credible information from trusted sources.

To improve the largely preventable conditions, we need both a combination of individual responsibility and health policy reforms. As this burden of chronic disease increases, there is lots that people can do to equip themselves with the knowledge and skills to make better-informed food choices. To plug the nutrition

gap that has emerged within healthcare, the British Society of Lifestyle Medicine has created a platform to provide information about evidence-based interventions focused on diet and nutrition. People can access this information by looking at www.bslm.org.uk and checking out the latest events and annual conference."

Cohort studies? Case series? Anecdotal? Eh?!?

You'll see 'scientific and clinical studies or evidence based' quite a few times in this book, so we thought we'd take a little tea break to teach you about the different levels and types. The 'hierarchy of evidence' is basically a league table for different types of scientific research.

Systematic reviews pool all relevant studies on a topic and try and reach a general conclusion based on all the studies available, which is why they are top dog. While bias is minimized, caution and a degree of critical thinking is still needed. They may look at several small studies and pool them together which would amplify any positive findings and magnify potential negatives. This can result in a misleading conclusion about a particular area. But when we talk about the individual studies reviewed within these reviews, Randomized Control Trials (RCTs) are widely considered the most reliable type of single study you can do BUT they too can have flaws...

Not only are RCTs good for monitoring what happens when you make people do something very specific, very differently, but they also RANDOMLY allocate participants to different groups for testing within the trial (intervention or no intervention) – this reduces the potential bias that may arise when selecting individuals for different groups. There are quite a few variables within this randomization and this all affects the reliability of the results. For example, do the participants know what they are receiving? The placebo effect is a real thing! That's why you will see single-blind (participants didn't know) or double blind (neither the researchers nor the participants know) when it comes to the intervention. The participants are then followed up after a set period of time, with the theory being that as the groups should be the same (on average), any differences between the groups will be due to the intervention (in theory...). When looking at an RCT, always check out who it has been funded by (e.g. a pharmaceutical company), study size and blinding.

heirarchy of evidence

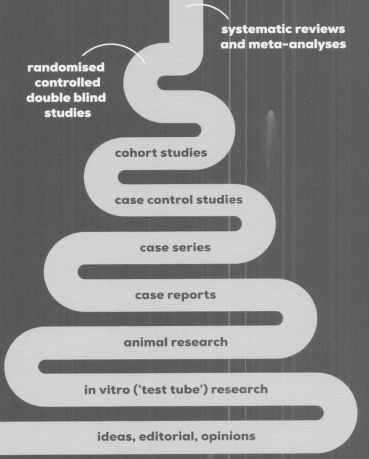

systematic reviews and meta-analyses

randomised controlled double blind studies

cohort studies

case control studies

case series

case reports

animal research

in vitro ('test tube') research

ideas, editorial, opinions

Why are RCTs so important? Well, they're often called interventions, as they are unusual, as scientists actually DO something to study participants and then look at what happens once they have introduced a change (e.g. a supplement or mindfulness). Other types of research design may involve a lab experiment in controlled surroundings (so not real life) or use surveys to observe people 'in the wild', and then try and draw links and conclusions between different treatments or risk factors and their outcomes. Hopefully this will make it all a bit easier to decipher and help you apply a critical eye to reviewing the evidence!

the gut and immunity

So, we know how the gut works, we know what affects it, and how it changes...

...but what impact does our gut have on the rest of us? We've included just a fraction of the complex connections our gut has with other parts of our body and how we move, sleep, and eat. Now we are handing the mic over to specialists in each field to help you understand more about your gut health!

First up on the stage, top immunologist Dr Jenna Macciochi to help explain the connection between your gut and immune system. Jenna has a PhD, is a lecturer, and was awarded a prestigious Presidential Fellowship to combine her personal interest in nutrition with the study of the immune system and, to complete her legendary status, she also has twins and is Scottish!

Before this journey, we thought the immune system was basically just about common colds and packets of Echinacea. How wrong we were...

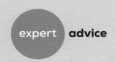
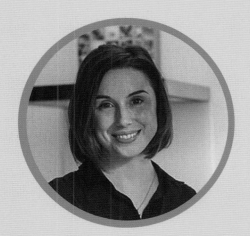

Dr Jenna Macciochi

"Most of us are aware that our immune system is our guardian against infection. But did you know our immune system has a complicated relationship with germs? Interacting with germs of all kinds – good and bad – is key to coaching and educating our immune system in how to behave properly and avoid unruly activities like allergies or autoimmune disease.

Bacteria educate our immune system from the moment we are born.

We know how important bacteria are for maintaining a normal immune system from experiments with germ-free laboratory mice born without any bacteria at all. The roots of this relationship lie in how you are born and nourished during the first five or so years of life. This is a key period of immune education that sets up your immune system for your long-term health.

Gut bacteria maintain a balanced immune system.

The immune system is complex and highly responsive to the world around us, so it's not surprising that there are many things that affect its function. And there is a good reason for this. Immunity is not hard-wired in our genes but educated by our environment and experiences. Much of this education takes place in our gut. It's true, and by now a familiar fact, that almost 70% of the entire immune system resides in the gut.

Throughout life, we are constantly exposed to new things via our gut, including foods, substances in our environment and, in some cases, germs. But thankfully, most people have a healthy immune system that handles all of these invading objects with ease. If they didn't, it would elicit a dangerous inflammatory response every time they tried a new food or visited a new environment with different types of germs, dust and dirt. The essential day-to-day task of your gut immune system is to maintain a balance between reacting to things that might hurt you and tolerating the things that won't, like good germs that we actually need. (Remember what we were talking about earlier – your gut keeps self and non-self apart, see page 25.) This is called 'oral tolerance'. Oral tolerance is when our immune system becomes trained to be unresponsive to something via the gut. It is extremely important to tolerate many of the harmless things we come across in our day-to-day lives, like the many components of food entering our gut. Much of this training happens in childhood, and our gut microbes help the process. Without it we can develop serious food allergies.

A diverse gut flora with many types of bacteria, fungi and other beneficial germs is a crucial part of this process. These germs teach the cells of the immune system that not everything is bad. And what happens in the gut doesn't stay in the gut but affects the functioning of the immune system throughout the body, influencing many aspects of health, including how immune cells seek out potential cancer cells, how well we recover from infections like flu and how well we control unruly inflammation from allergies and autoimmunity."

"A diverse gut flora is the healthiest.

And we are all unique. Most bacteria are beneficial, but some are responsible for making us unwell. An unhealthy microbiota might look different in different people, but they all have one thing in common: a lack of diversity. A diverse microbiota is more likely to bounce back from unhealthy fluctuations in diet and withstand outside intruders, and this means a much more tolerant and well-regulated immune system."

immunity and the gut

your body's ability to fight diseases and infections

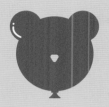

gut microbes educate and support your immune system – immunity is made not born – early years are crucial!

"hello and welcome to microbe middle school"

houses 70% of your immune system

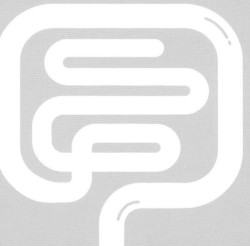

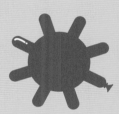

when your microbes are acting out of sorts they can disrupt your immune system

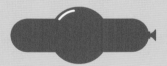

inflammation is part of your immune response but when it is prolonged, it can negatively impact your gut and increase your risk of certain conditions

impacted by stress, pathogens, modern living, allergies, medication, and sleep

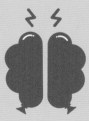

your immune system isn't static, its cells travel all over your body to where they are needed

"all aboard the bloodstream express"

How do you keep your gut microbes (and your immune system) healthy?

Decreased exposure to infections in early life through improved hygiene was originally thought to be the main way our immunity was 'trained'. But rather than being too clean, the most important change in our environment that leaves us open to allergies is the loss of contact with our 'old friends' – the many harmless microbes in us, on us and around us from birth. So how does our immune system see these 'old friends'?

The birthing process sets off the most radical transformation – a tsunami of good gut microbes colonizes the (relatively) sterile baby as it enters the world. So, receiving foundational microbes with the potential to educate immunity starts with your mother. These initial microbes were inherited from their mother, and so on. The next thing is breast milk, which comes conveniently packaged as a food source not just for the baby but for their gut bugs too. In contrast, caesarean sections and formula feeding have been shown to have a negative impact on our gut bacterial species. While standard infant formula doesn't contain these natural milk prebiotics, some formulas now have different added beneficial prebiotics. Apart from our mothers and our diets, we also obtain our microbes from our environment. So regardless of how you were born, there is plenty you can do to change your gut microbes for the better.

You cannot control how you came into the world, but there are some things you can do to improve your gut health:

- Get more plant diversity in your diet. The fibre in plants passes through the digestive system until it reaches the colon, where it provides the fodder for your gut microbes. When they chow down fibre, they release a load of powerful immune-nourishing molecules.

- Get out, get dirty and rewild your microbes. You might have heard that we are 'too clean', which is bad for our health. As well as getting microbes via our diets, we also get them from our environment. Dirt is good. Disconnection from nature is not.

Modern urban life is low on microbial diversity and discourages contact with beneficial environmental microbiomes. For those of us not living in the countryside, our immune systems may be missing out on those environmental microbes. Ensure a regular counterbalance, like spending time in a garden, regularly stepping out into the countryside or a park, doing some gardening (even if it's just your windowsill or going to a community allotment). The more contact we have with dirt and natural environments, the more we let their microbiomes infiltrate and nurture our own.

- Be mindful of antibiotics. Unfortunately, antibiotics sweep through the gut and kill off both unfriendly and beneficial gut microbes. It is best to try to avoid them where possible, but sometimes you need to take a course of antibiotics. After you've finished the treatment, the beneficial gut microbes and the unfriendly ones slowly rebuild and, if all goes well, they come back into balance. But, it takes time, and they don't always colonize in harmony. Probiotics may help your gut recover its balance faster. Consuming probiotics reduces the incidence of diarrhoea associated with taking antibiotics, which affects around 30% of people. However, there aren't enough studies of any one particular probiotic to say conclusively which one works and which one doesn't. Different strains do different things. Follow the tips for general good gut health on pages 98–103.

- Take your time – probably one of the biggest hurdles in our busy modern lives. Planning regular meals can be helpful for reducing stress and making sure that you don't overeat at your next meal, both of which are bad news for your beneficial microbes. Excessive stress can negatively impact your immune system too.

the gut-brain

We've always known our gut and brain are linked, we get butterflies in our stomachs if we see the person we fancy, or have to run to the loo when know we have to speak publicly. But did you know the conversation happens both ways?

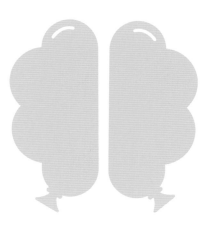

gut–brain axis tennis match

To introduce this section, we have none other than the champions of the gut–brain axis themselves: John Cryan and Ted Dinan, of APC Microbiome Ireland, University College Cork, and our hero of all things 'brain', Kimberley Wilson, in a game of intellectual tag-team tennis.

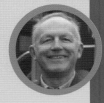

player(s) 1

Ted is a Cork psychiatrist. In 2019 he was ranked by Expertscape as the number one global expert on the microbiota and also listed in the top one hundred Global Makers and Mavericks. He has published over 500 papers and is co-author, with John, of the bestseller *The Psychobiotic Revolution*. John is a senior editor of *Neuropharmacology and Nutritional Neuroscience*, editor of the *British Journal of Pharmacology* and the list is endless for the amount of peer-reviewed papers he's written and how much he's been cited. He was also included in the 2014 list of the 'World's Most Influential Scientific Minds' – very cool!

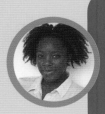

player 2

Kimberley Wilson is a chartered psychologist and one of the best founts of knowledge we know – her book *How to Build a Healthy Brain* is a MUST-READ. She also came second on *The Great British Bake Off* (!!).

Kimberley Wilson for the opening serve...

"We need to get away from the idea that the brain and the body are separate entities that simply communicate with each other. Not only does this not make any sense (how is the brain kept alive if not through the oxygen, nutrients and energy supplied by the body?), but it has slowed down the progress of medical and psychiatric research and treatment for decades."

A strong return up next from John and Ted...

"To have 'a gut feeling' is a term familiar to most people and translates equally well in almost all languages. Given this fact, it is perhaps surprising that the view that our gut may influence our brain has only gained traction with scientists in recent times. Study of the gut–brain axis has become one of the most hotly researched areas in biology over the past twenty years. We now know that microbes within our gut have a profound effect on how our brain functions. The majority of microbes in our gut live in the large intestine. The average adult has about 1kg of microbes in the intestine, which is approximately the same weight as our brains. These microbes are fed by us and, in turn, they produce molecules that our brains require. We cannot survive without our microbes and they cannot survive without us. We have evolved with microbes and would not function properly without them. It now seems strange that for so many decades we viewed the gut microbiota as consisting of commensal microbes that did us no harm but were of little benefit. How wrong we were!"

Kimberley to deploy vagus nerve shot for the next point...

"The beautiful, wandering vagus nerve is a real multitasker. Going from your brain to your gut and connecting through all of your major organs along the way, the vagus nerve is the major structural component of the gut–brain axis. But it doesn't stop there – the vagus nerve is also the main structural feature of the parasympathetic nervous system (PSNS). The PSNS is the flip-side of your 'fight or flight' response, aka your sympathetic nervous system (SNS). While the SNS is responsible for preparing your body for action – increasing blood pressure and breathing rate, shutting down digestion to make more oxygen carried in your blood available to your arms and legs etc. – the PSNS returns the body to a state of calm and rest. This is the reason that IBS symptoms are so often triggered by stress and why you should avoid trying to eat when you are agitated or in a rush; you won't be able to digest your food properly."

The microbial ball serve from John and Ted...

"How do gut microbes and the brain communicate? There are several parallel routes of communication. The long, meandering vagus nerve sends signals in both directions from gut to brain and brain to gut. Some bacteria cannot signal to the brain if this nerve is damaged. Another important communication pathway is the production by bacteria of short-chain fatty acids (SCFA), such as butyrate (see pages 54–55). These are important molecules for generating energy but can also impact how the genes within our cells work. Microbes also produce tryptophan, which is the building block for serotonin (5-HT) in our brains. Serotonin plays a key role in regulating sleep and mood, and most medications used for treating depression act upon this chemical. Our research has shown that the gut microbes of those suffering from depression differ from the microbes of healthy individuals. To maintain a healthy state of mind we need to look after our gut microbes."

Kimberley's final volley...

"There is another important way that the gut communicates with the brain and that is through the immune system. The majority of the body's immune cells are found around the gut. This makes sense because food is one of the most common carriers of harmful bugs (like spoiled meat or a dodgy prawn sarnie left out for too long) and your body wants to be ready. Inflammation is the immune system's response to illness or injury. When a pathogen, like a virus or harmful bacteria, is detected, immune cells kick into action, releasing signalling molecules and powerful chemicals to kill off the threat. Once the threat is under control, the inflammation will normally die down. However, lifestyle factors such as diet can also influence immunity.

If you are not getting enough fibre in your diet, your gut microbes effectively begin to starve. Faced with this situation, they turn to a backup fuel source called mucin. Unfortunately, mucin forms the protective mucus layer that coats the inside of your gut (see page 25). If your gut microbes eat through it, the tight cell junctions in the gut wall can open and become permeable. When this happens, bacteria and food molecules from the gut can enter the bloodstream. Seeing these intruders in the bloodstream, your immune system launches an attack and if this goes on for a long time you are likely to be in a state of chronic inflammation. As this blood flows through the brain it can trigger neuroinflammation, which is associated with an increased risk of a range of mental health conditions, including depression, bipolar disorder and Alzheimer's disease. So, feeding your gut with plenty of diverse sources of fibre is actually a crucial part of a brain-healthy lifestyle."

And there we have it, a physical and chemical (and an immunity bonus) match of the best minds. Now for the post-match breakdown and takeaways (the factual kind, not a post-match pint).

gut- brain axis

Amygdala may be influenced by your gut microbiome – more activity here may increase risk of anxiety.

physically connected by the vagus nerve

chemically connected by neurotransmitters

Different types of microbes and their by-products, may increase or decrease risk of mental health conditions, like anxiety and depression.

What goes on in the gut does not stay in the gut. Inflammation in the gut can affect the brain.

neurotransmitters

serotonin
Happiness, linked to body clock and anxiety (if levels low). Found mostly in the gut, utilised by the brain.

gaba
Calming, moderates anxiety, made in brain and gut. Gaba receptors in brain and the gut. low levels increase risk of anxiety.

dopamine
Motivator, pleasure, memory, mood and sleep. Produced in the gut. low levels increase risk of anxiety.

the gut
and stress

**Stress is often a driver behind many
different gut symptoms...**

...and so it makes sense to learn how to manage stress and calm down (easier said than done – we know). Doing activities that relax you, such as deep breathing, yoga and meditation (or even having a laugh with a mate) encourages your body to activate the parasympathetic nervous system (rest and digest) instead of the sympathetic nervous system (fight or flight). Being in fight or flight mode is a good thing, providing it activates at the right time, but not if you are trying to digest food or need to get to sleep.

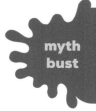

**myth
bust**

"De-stressing must be about gong baths and candles."

TAKEAWAY
Take three deep breaths before eating, enough to switch to rest-and-digest mode.

stress and your gut

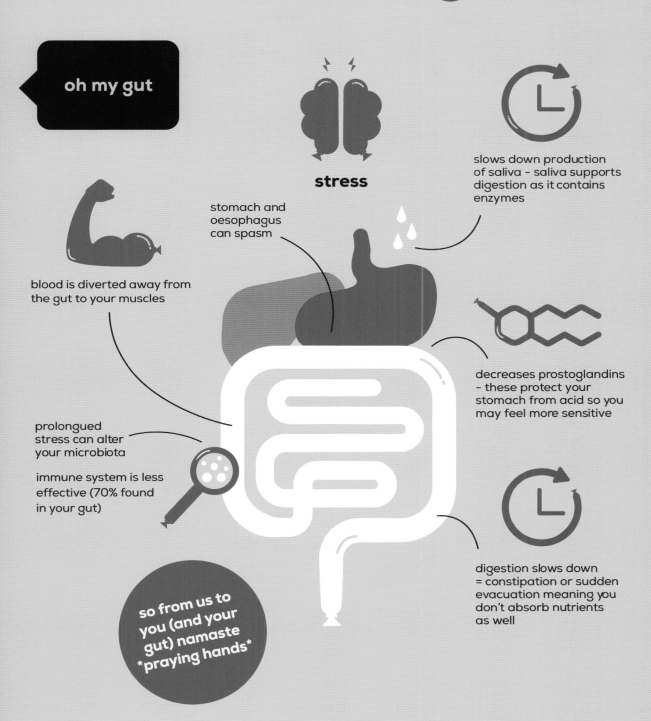

oh my gut

stress

slows down production of saliva - saliva supports digestion as it contains enzymes

stomach and oesophagus can spasm

blood is diverted away from the gut to your muscles

decreases prostoglandins – these protect your stomach from acid so you may feel more sensitive

prolongued stress can alter your microbiota

immune system is less effective (70% found in your gut)

digestion slows down = constipation or sudden evacuation meaning you don't absorb nutrients as well

so from us to you (and your gut) namaste *praying hands*

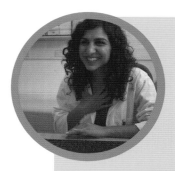

breathwork
with dr rabia

Before we'd tried breathwork we were like, 'breath-what? We do that anyway, surely?'

Then we did a session with Dr Rabia, a gastroenterologist and a yoga instructor (what a combo!) and we knew we had to share her magic with you...

"Take a deep inhale...
pause at the top...
exhale out through the mouth."

"What is the power of conscious breathing? What does it have to do with your digestive health? Our story begins with the close relationship between your nervous system and gut: as we have now understood, the two are married from birth. Modern life favours a swing towards 'fight or flight' mode (the so-called sympathetic drive), which can dictate our eating habits, pain threshold and anxiety levels. The rhythm of our body in times of stress – even if we are not fully aware of it – often involves shallow and rapid breathing, primarily in the upper chest, and is associated with an increased heart rate. This synchrony of heart rate and breathing is called Respiratory Sinus Arrhythmia (RSA) and is part of the normal, automatic processes governed by our trusty vagus nerve (see page 43). Therefore, this pattern also reflects the tone in our belly, as the vagus nerve communicates the motion within our gut.

But how can we nudge the conversation in the other direction? Put simply, we can influence vagus nerve activity by consciously altering the rate and depth of our breathing. RSA is a signal that appears like waves on the ocean – and you are steering the ship. Interestingly, this surrogate marker of vagal nerve activity is most influenced during the exhalation portion of our breath cycle. Extending your exhale just slightly longer than your inhale and slowing down your rate of breathing provides a kind of massage for the vagus nerve. This can correspond to better synchronization between the brain and gut by enabling us to regulate our stress levels and our perception of symptoms.

If you were guided by my instruction at the start to indulge in a single, deep sigh (feel free to do it again and observe), you will notice that the very act of simply bringing awareness to your breath provides a conscious shift to slow down and check in. We all naturally breathe at different rates, oscillating depending on the circumstance. My first tip is to notice what your breathing is telling you right now. With this awareness, bring your attention and breath down into your belly and relax the muscles of the abdominal wall. We do this by engaging the large, sling-like muscle at the bottom of the ribs: our diaphragm. When the movement of this muscle is out of sync with the muscles in our belly, it can exacerbate bloating and discomfort. So, my second tip is to soften the belly: allow the rise and fall of each breath to occur from this space. In many ways the journey to ease, comfort and control begins with a single, deep breath."

the gut
and sleep

Anecdotally (no science, just us!), we noticed that when we were touring and dj-ing with 1am set times it wasn't great on our guts...

...so the gut and sleep is an area of research we wanted to get our noses right into as 1 in 5 of us don't get enough sleep and it can play a huge role in our health.

The neurotransmitters produced (remember them from the tennis match, pages 41–44) and released by your gut microbes, such as dopamine, serotonin (the precursor to melatonin – your sleep-regulating hormone) and GABA, all impact your sleep. Sleep has the ability to affect all areas of your health, including your gut, immune system and mental health. All of this is part of the gut–brain axis – it's all linked – almost like we were made this way for a reason.

Shift work, different time zones, poor-quality sleep and/or late or irregular bedtimes can disrupt your circadian rhythm and affect the health of your microbes and their composition. Indeed, your microbes have their own circadian rhythm and have different functions at different times of the day. Think of your microbes as hotel workers: you have your regular kitchen staff making breakfast, lunch and dinner and then, come late evening, the room service chefs take over, often with a different menu and different roles to fulfil. So, if you suddenly start demanding lunch at midnight, you can see how your microbes might be

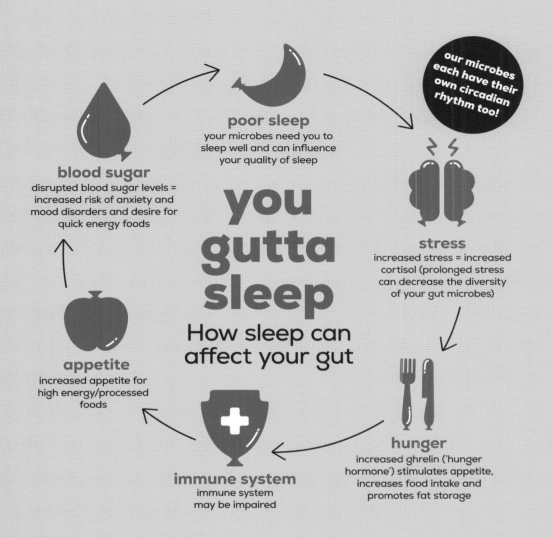

you gutta sleep
How sleep can affect your gut

poor sleep
your microbes need you to sleep well and can influence your quality of sleep

our microbes each have their own circadian rhythm too!

stress
increased stress = increased cortisol (prolonged stress can decrease the diversity of your gut microbes)

hunger
increased ghrelin ('hunger hormone') stimulates appetite, increases food intake and promotes fat storage

immune system
immune system may be impaired

appetite
increased appetite for high energy/processed foods

blood sugar
disrupted blood sugar levels = increased risk of anxiety and mood disorders and desire for quick energy foods

a bit confused. This kind of explains why when you're on holiday in an actual hotel in a different time zone, you have a funny feeling for the first couple of days, which will also be affecting your gut microbes' hotel, too.

Research shows that if you have better-quality sleep, your cognitive function is increased (bye-bye brain fog!) and you are more likely to have a greater number of beneficial microbes in your gut. Caveat: we still need more information about the link between cognitive function, the microbiota and sleep to conclusively prove this relationship.

As The Rock once said in a popular Disney movie, let's turn our attention from lessons to 'takeaways'.

sleep hygiene

We aren't just talking about a clean bed here (although that can help too!). A little routine that you do every night can help set you up for consistent and optimal sleep which supports you and your microbes, and can make all the difference. We had always pooh-poohed (you don't get away from the poo chat for long!) this before as we had such extreme night patterns, but then we started it and ZZZZZZzzzzzzzzzzzzzzzzz...

- Set a sleep and wake time and try to stick to them – this helps your circadian rhythm.

- Limit your use of screens in the hour or so before bed. Dim your lights and avoid those horror films. There's a setting on most phones that will automatically reduce the light from a certain time in case you forget!

- Take time to wind down from your day. Read or listen to a book, meditate, enjoy a warm bath, do some gentle stretching – whatever works for you.

- Keep your phone out of your bedroom and get an alarm clock (hello old-school!) if you rely on your phone's alarm.

- Avoid stimulants before bedtime, such as caffeine and nicotine. A note on caffeine: genetics, age and weight will determine how quickly your body metabolizes caffeine. It has a half-life of 5–7 hours, which means it isn't just about avoiding caffeine in the evening, but also later in the afternoon too.

- Make your bedroom a relaxing place for sleep. Keep it cool and dark and minimize distractions.

- Avoid overindulging before bedtime as this can disrupt your sleep and microbes (think about the hotel workers, see page 50–51).

You'll find what works for you; we always find that writing our to-do lists for the next day can empty our heads a bit and leave space for the nice dreams to come in.

the gut
and exercise

We know that what you eat can have a big impact on your gut. But did you know that exercise has the ability to change your gut microbes independently of anything else? Sounds like an easy win to us. Over to our head of nutrition and all-round brainbox Kristy Coleman for this one...

"Exercise can help change both the composition of your gut microbes and how they function, and that's even without having to eat some funky fermented foods. But it really depends on the type of exercise you are doing and how hard you are doing it, so it's not that simple (as you're probably starting to gather).

When the microbes in your gut ferment fibre, they produce short-chain fatty acids, one of which is called butyrate. Butyrate is fuel for your gut cells and keeps your gut lining healthy, helps regulate your immune system and supports other functions too (clever clogs!). Some studies even suggest it may play a role in sleep, supporting immune function and helping with diarrhoea control. So, in short, we want our microbes to be producing it and have the right ones there in the first place to do so. Research has shown that just five weeks of exercise increased the number of microbes producing butyrate. More research on rugby players showed that they had forty different types of bacteria compared to those who were sedentary, aka coach potatoes (scientific term)! Studies in women have shown that those who did at least three hours of exercise per week had increased levels of certain bacteria known to produce butyrate and had high amounts of a bacteria called *Akkermansia muciniphila* (which lives in your mucus lining, see page 25), which is associated with a lean BMI.

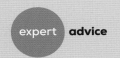
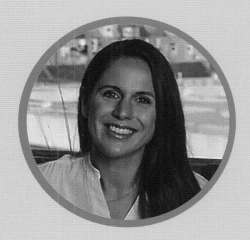

So, does this mean you can eat what you want providing you exercise? If only it was that simple. Everybody is different, so we can't be sure what types of exercise will do what, and it's difficult to control all aspects of a study to know what is having the impact on your microbes. Sedentary people are also more likely to eat less healthily than those who are active, so that will have an impact too. BUT the overall consensus is that exercise is important for a healthy gut, whether it's hitting the dance floor or a gym class – your gut likes you to move. Just don't go too hard on high-intensity sessions, as this can cause stress, which we know has a knock-on effect on your gut and immune system."

Kristy Coleman

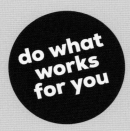

do what works for you

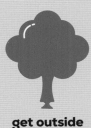

get outside and move

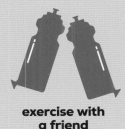

exercise with a friend

movement and the gut

stand up, or walk & talk

put on some tunes & dance

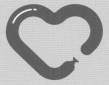

do something you enjoy

like goldilocks, do what's 'just right' for you

the gut and skin

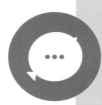

Another expert who's constantly on our speed dial is consultant dermatologist, author of *The Skincare Bible,* and all-round queen Anjali Mahto. Our conversations with her go something like this:

"Anjali, which moisturizer has SPF in it?"
"Anjali, do chemical peels really work?"
"Anjali, *insert pic* what is this on my face?"
"Anjali, we've been asked about acne again–
please can you do another blog post?"

You can see where this is going, so we knew we had to get her take on the gut and skin. It's a super exciting area of research, so we need a measured head to walk us through it...

"It has long been recognized in medical literature that many skin disorders are more common in those with gut issues and vice versa. Data shows that rosacea is associated with small intestinal bacterial overgrowth (SIBO), and treatment of this can improve the primary skin condition. Conversely, those who suffer with inflammatory bowel disease (IBD) are at higher risk of developing inflammatory skin conditions such as psoriasis.

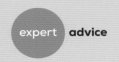

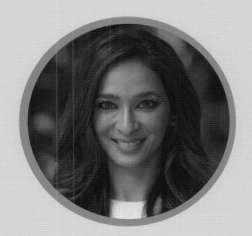

Anjali Mahto

So how do the gut and skin communicate with each other? While this area of research is growing rapidly, there are a number of proposed mechanisms by which the gut and skin are understood to interact:

Microbial imbalance (see dysbiosis on page 272) in the gut may cause the production of a number of molecules or metabolites (some produced by your microbes) that can access the circulation and accumulate in distant sites, such as the skin, having a negative impact.

Disturbed gut barrier (see page 25) may result in gut bacteria themselves entering the circulation and travelling to the skin. Supportive data suggests bacterial DNA of intestinal origin has been found in the blood circulation of those with psoriasis, meaning it probably got there by escaping through the wall of the gut.

Dysbiosis or gut imbalance may interfere with the immune response in skin disease by increasing the activity of certain immune cells that drive inflammation (more on inflammation later, see page 44).

Changes in the gut microbiome may directly affect or induce changes in resident microbes in the skin (or skin microbiome).

Although there are multiple pathways allowing for gut–skin interaction, there is much we still do not understand. Gut microbiota alterations have been implicated in common skin conditions such as acne, eczema and psoriasis. However, as these ailments have multifactorial triggers for development, including interaction between genetics and the environment, it is difficult to say how gut microbiota interactions directly fit into the complex picture of disease development.

What we do know, though, is that eating well for your skin is no different to eating well for your general health. While skin disease should not be treated with diet alone where validated therapeutic options exist, there is no doubt that diet has a part to play as a piece of the wider puzzle. Diet can influence the course of skin disease, have a preventative role in disease development and affect future health outcomes. Both short- and long-term dietary habits can alter gut microbial composition and have the potential to affect skin in both health and disease states. This may in part be achieved by sustained eating patterns incorporating:

- essential fatty acids, found most abundantly in oily fish and in walnuts and flaxseeds for plant-based sources.

- carotenoids, found in foods like apricots, watermelon, asparagus, carrots, squash, sweet potato and tomatoes (and plenty more).

- vitamin C – think berries, citrus fruits, sweet and white potatoes and broccoli.

- vitamin E, found in foods like sunflower seeds, almonds, hazelnuts, pine nuts (need an excuse for pesto), peanuts, salmon and avocado.

- minerals, including copper, zinc and selenium found in nuts, seeds, dark leafy greens, shellfish, wholegrains and oily fish.

- polyphenols, essentially lots of colourful plant-based foods.

- fermented foods (jump to page 102)."

"Early data shows there may be a role for probiotic supplementation, but it remains to be seen how effective this approach will be. As we discover and understand more about the pathways by which the gut and skin communicate with each other, we may in future be able to target certain skin conditions by manipulating the gut microbiome."

Watch this space!

pre- and probiotics

Before we get on to the *how*, we need to take a quick trip back to school (not over yet!), to the fun of the science labs and Bunsen burners, to learn about pre- and probiotics. What's the difference? Although the names are confusingly similar, prebiotics and probiotics are actually very different, and you need a good mix of both to keep your gut happy.

The WHO defines a probiotic as 'a live micro-organism which, when eaten or drunk in adequate amounts, confers a health benefit on the host' (you!). Probiotics can be in food or supplement form but not all probiotics are created equal – different strains have different effects, and some might have no effect at all; it all depends on the individual. Science is still learning exactly how different strains work, so watch this space.

Foods containing probiotics include live yogurt, kimchi, sauerkraut, kefir, miso and kombucha. Try to get a mix of different types across the course of your week; we like to experiment and make our own sauerkraut, as it's cheap and super easy. (More about how to do this later, see page 256.)

Here's a little picture to put in your pocket to read the gobbledegook of supplement packaging. We've made it super simple for you.

1. **Ingredients:** all ingredients (not just cultures) and allergens in order of weight
2. **Total Active Cell Count:** colony forming units (CFU) – number of live cultures (usually at time of manufacture). CFU for total count but for each strain better

3. **Bacterial Strains:** need all three bits:
   1. Lactobaccilus = genus
   2. Rhamanos = species
   3. XYZ = designation of strains / different designations of a strain will have a different role
4. **Use:** how to use
5. **Storage:** how to store: some may need to be kept cold, others somewhere cool and dry
6. **Claims:** approved claims for the amount of cultures in probiotic – must be scientifically evaluated and approved by EFSA

probi-what-ics?

1 **ingredients:**
Capsule, Live Cultures, Allergens

2 **total active cell count:**
10^9 5.0 Colony Forming Units (CFU)
Each capsule: 1.25^1 CFU

3 **bacterial strains:**
ADF
Z3
XY4

4 **use:**
Dose

best before:
00/00/00

5 **storage:**
How, out of reach of children. Not substitute for varied diet.

company:
Probiotic King & Queen

6 **claims:**
Supports xyz.

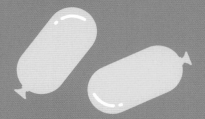

When it comes to supplements, it's very difficult to decipher fact versus expensive marketing jargon to work out which products are efficacious. We'd advise focusing on the different strains of bacteria in a product and researching a bit about what that particular strain is good for.

prebiotics: 25 years on

Now we've got probiotics covered, what about prebiotics? Prebiotics are a specific type of fibre and the food for good bacteria. Great food sources of prebiotics include onions, garlic, leeks, chicory, bananas (the unripe green ones that nobody wants), asparagus, artichokes, olives, plums and apples, plus wholegrains like bran and nuts like almonds.

As a nice break in the science, we wanted to share this little anecdote with you. Professor Glenn Gibson is a microbiology professor at the University of Reading. He has worked in university or research institutes since he left home (Horden, Co. Durham) in 1979 and has published almost 500 research papers, supervised 75 PhD students, and carried out 140 research contracts. He started the research on prebiotics improving gut health and has studied people's faeces for over 30 years. He has no sense of smell ;)

Glenn is the founding father of prebiotics; we met him recently and loved hearing how these breakthroughs came about from the man behind the science. We couldn't write a book about gut health and not include his story, so grab a beer and pull up a seat at the bar with him, where this story is set...

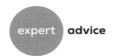

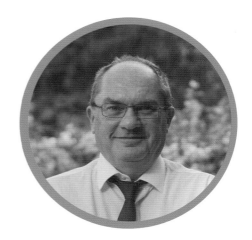

Professor Glenn Gibson

"I can remember three things about my academic life in the 1990s...

1. Working with John Cummings in his gut group at the MRC-Dunn Human Nutrition Unit at the University of Cambridge (the other microbiologist being my sadly missed friend George Macfarlane).

2. My first PhD student being Xin Wang.

3. Not suffering the major hair loss that my subsequent working career has caused.

As part of Xin's research, I was introduced to Marcel Roberfroid. Like John, he is a real gentleman as well as an excellent scientist. Marcel was a consultant to the company who sponsored Xin's project, known as Raffinerie Tirlemontoise, then Orafti (much easier to say), now Beneo-Institute. The research was on using inulin to boost beneficial bacteria in the gut, using laboratory fermenters and two human studies. This was before the molecular revolution hit gut microbiology and I remember poor Xin having to biochemically characterize every colony that had grown on thousands of supposedly selective Petri dish agars.

Marcel and I would have frequent meetings in the Scandic Crown Hotel, near Victoria, when he was in London – in the bar of course! At one of these, we chatted about how the inulin was a bit like a probiotic, in that it was changing the gut bacteriology for the better, but it did not have the survival issues that using live microbes in the diet could have. We decided to write a review on the research, and other similar studies, showing how carbohydrates could selectively fortify beneficial gut bacteria like bifidobacteria. I suggested we should give this concept a name and we agreed to think about possibilities. I went home and started drafting the review. About two hours later I sent it to Marcel, who then turned my words into something more resembling science and he drafted the figures (one of which was in colour – unheard of back then!). We finished in it a few days.

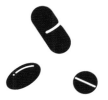

"Prebiotics have safely helped to improve the gut health of people and animals."

Then the argument started about the concept name. I favoured 'parabiotics'. This was driven by one fact alone. At the time, *MASH* (Mobile Army Surgical Hospital) was a popular comedy programme in the UK. It was an American series, set in the Korean War, featuring paramedics, and these were people who helped medics. So, a 'parabiotic' would help biotics – right? Wrong, according to Marcel, who instead proposed 'prebiotics'. We went with that and called the paper 'Dietary Modulation of the Human Colonic Microbiota – Introducing the Concept of Prebiotics'. It was published in *The Journal of Nutrition* in 1995.

Little did we know the impact that a review that took only a few hours to write would have. I can't comment on the quality because I have not read it since publication (in common with the rest of my embarrassing writing). Marcel did all the good bits in there anyway.

25 years later, the following still amazes me:

- The prebiotic concept is now the subject of several conferences, meetings and workshops each year.

- New prebiotic dietary products have arisen, as well as variations of existing ones.

- Prebiotics is a term often used by consumers – this is unusual in the field of microbiology, which is plagued by jargon.

- I've seen 'prebiotics' written on numerous product boxes and even heard it on many TV and radio adverts.

- In 2018, Yeung et al. (*Food Chemistry* 269, 455–465) reported that our review was the most highly cited of any functional foods papers ever published, with 3,797 citations at that time. This is madness!

- There are now 3,000–5,000 research papers on prebiotics (depending on which website you look at).

- Prebiotics have a value of $3–16 billion worldwide (depending on which website you look at).

- There is a predicted 11–15% economic and scientific rise in this subject over the next five years (depending on which website you look at).

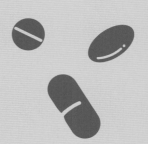

I've always known that the most productive research originates in a bar... but all of this pales into insignificance compared to the instances where prebiotics have safely helped to improve the gut health of people and animals, as they were intended to.

P.S. One common comment I get is, "You should have called it something else". My usual reply is, "Such as?" That usually elicits silence – but I still think I was right with 'parabiotics'...

P.P.S. It is not all plain sailing: in 2004 *The Journal of Nutrition* rejected our follow-up review updating the concept."

What a guy!

We can't wait to see where he takes the research next.

i've gutta problem

When we originally set up The Gut Stuff we just wanted to shout from the rooftops about all the cool science around the microbiome we were learning about, but as we delved in, we realized just how many people were living with digestive issues, and, even more worryingly, in silence...

Most of us hide behind 'the poo taboo' and lose track into adulthood of how fascinated we are by the stuff as kids. With babies (and puppies!), we always use poos as an indication of how they're getting on (we have proper doggy plopsy inspections in our garden with our puppy!). We need to re-ignite this curiosity and perform some close monitoring on ourselves.

when to worry about your gut

In this next section we'll be teaching you how to peek before you flush, what to look out for and how to monitor other symptoms, such as bloating, farting, pain and all the other uncomfortable stuff, to help you spot the signs that something might be up. One in four of us has a digestive symptom at any one time, and these can be confusing as they often overlap. This section should help tease out the issues and teach you how to tune in.

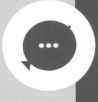

We knew we'd need a VERY safe pair of hands for this – Sophie Medlin is a registered dietitian and co-founder of CityDietitians. Sophie has been a specialist colorectal dietitian for over ten years. She works with patients who have conditions such as Crohn's disease, ulcerative colitis, bowel cancer and diverticular disease to help improve their nutritional status and their experience of eating, so you can see why we had to have her for this chapter. Take it away Soph...

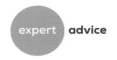

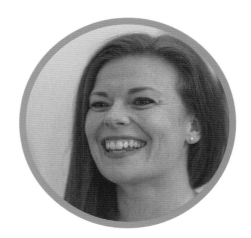

Sophie Medlin

"This is what you need to look out for in case something isn't right. First of all, let's cover what is 'normal':

Frequency – Anything from having your bowels open three times per day to three times per week.

Colour – Normal, healthy stools are usually a dark brown colour like chocolate or conkers. There are some exceptions to this rule, with certain foods, for example, when you eat beetroot, sometimes they can turn a funky purple colour!

Consistency – A normal stool is between a three and a four on the Bristol Stool Form Scale (see page 71). This means that it holds together like a sausage, but it shouldn't cause pain or require a lot of straining to get it out.

Wind – Having wind is completely normal and the amount will vary from day to day, depending on what you've eaten and how much exercise you've done, for example.

Pain – Occasional, mild stomach ache that passes when your bowels open is not a concern.

Bloating – Mild bloating after eating certain foods or a big meal is common and is not a cause for concern unless it is bothering you or it is particularly frequent."

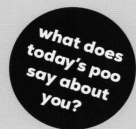

the gut stuff stool chart

what does today's poo say about you?

1 like nuts, hard to poop out – ouch!

2 like a bumpy chocolate bar

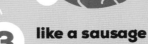

3 like a sausage but with cracks

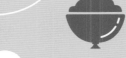

4 like a banana, smooth and soft

5 soft blobs with edges – like lumps of porridge

6 fluffy pieces like mushy peas with ragged edges

does yours sink or swim?

7 so runny, it's not funny

The first step in diagnosing bowel problems is usually a blood or stool test so there is nothing to be nervous about when you're speaking to your doctor for the first time.

Your stools (the technical term for poo) come in all kinds of shades, shapes and sizes and sometimes come more frequently and sometimes not as often. Because we're not very good at talking about our poo, we sometimes worry unnecessarily and sometimes we don't tell our doctor things that they do need to know.

Your body is really clever at giving you clues when something isn't right. To understand the symptoms, you need to talk to your doctor about them. Remember, it's about YOU, and we're all individual, so it's important to understand there's no right or wrong – it's about tuning in and getting to know your patterns so you can tell when something is up.

Things to report!

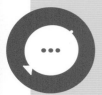

How often you go
Anywhere between three times a day and once every three days is considered normal.

Changes to your stools
On different days and sometimes at different times of the month (if you have periods), your stool might change for a few days. This is completely normal. If you notice a change in your poo that lasts for more than a couple of weeks it is important to tell your doctor. Even if this means that you notice that you're suddenly less constipated and you don't know why.

Red flags!

If you experience any of these symptoms, you need to speak to your doctor:

Blood in your stools
If there is blood on the toilet paper, also check to see if there is any blood mixed in with the poo. This will help your doctor to know where the blood is coming from. Old blood in your stool looks like black tar, so keep an eye out for that too.

Persistent pain or bloating
This means pain and bloating that doesn't go away when you pass a stool or pass wind, or if you are woken up in the night with pain and bloating. Also, if you notice that you get pain and bloating that builds up and that you have a sudden great urgency to go; then when you do go, you pass hard stools followed by liquid.

Sand- or yellow-coloured stools
Stools that are a pale sandy colour or are yellow need to be investigated. If you're losing weight as well, make sure you tell your doctor that too. Poo that is green usually means you've got a stomach bug and generally lasts a few days. Any longer, seek help from a doctor.

Stools that are frothy, foamy or contain mucus

These symptoms can happen after a bug or if you've eaten something that didn't agree with you, but if it doesn't settle down in a few days, chat to your doctor.

Stools that don't flush away

Stools that regularly block the toilet, or that float and take several flushes to get rid of, need to be reported, particularly if you can see undigested food in your stools. You also need to let your doctor know if you can see an oily residue in the toilet after you've been. Usually this will be yellowish in colour.

Stools that smell very bad

The question we ask patients is: "do you think your stools are particularly foul smelling?". If they are regularly smellier than you think they should be but you're already eating a healthy diet, then it is worth getting this checked out.

Other things!

If you notice your poo getting thin and pencil-like or ribbony, then that needs to be reported to your doctor, as does 'wet wind', which is the technical term for following through when you think it was just a fart! Reporting all these symptoms can help your doctor or dietitian to decide which tests you might need to diagnose your problem. Some of these symptoms suggest a problem with how you are absorbing your food. Some suggest a problem with how your stools are moving along the bowel and some suggest inflammation. Whatever is going on in there, it needs to be investigated and your doctor might not always know the right questions to ask, so make sure you're ready to share the details. Think about keeping a food and symptom diary to share if you find it hard to say the words out loud.

other sh*t you should know

You may never have considered how you poo, but toddlers have got it right with this potty business.

Sitting on a Western-style toilet means your puborectalis muscle contracts, which means your rectum is tight, making evacuation of poo difficult, straining and putting pressure on your pelvic floor.

Squatting with your feet on a 20–30cm high step relaxes your puborectalis muscle (allowing your rectum to open properly), making it easier for poo to evacuate and preventing straining.

Get yourself a step or a box (or even a pile of books!) to put near your toilet and gut in POOsition!

how do you poo?

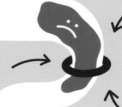

puborectalis
muscle contracts
squeezing rectum

increases straining and
pelvic floor pressure

kinda like
a water
flume with
a kink in it

squatting

eg. feet on step
20–30cm high

protects
nerves

puborectalis
muscle relaxes
allowing rectum
to open

prevents
straining

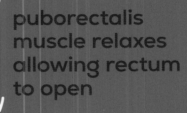

analrectal
straightened

gut in
POOsition!

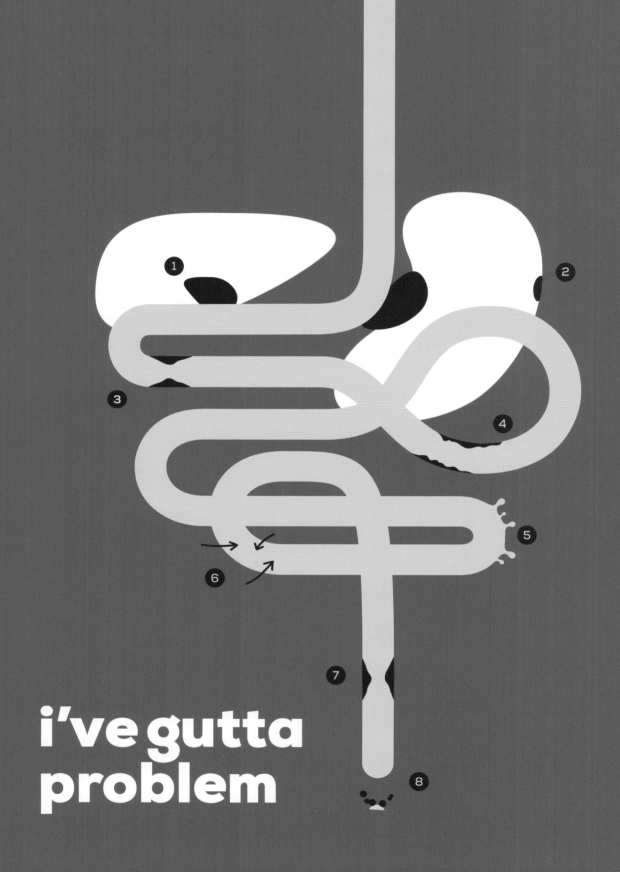

i've gutta
problem

1. Stools that are pale in colour, foul smelling, frothy, oily or difficult to flush away are associated with not absorbing all your food properly. Sometimes this is linked to your gall bladder, bile metabolism or pancreas.

2. Stools that are black and tar-like are sometimes caused by blood that is coming from something higher up in your gut, such as stomach ulcers.

3. Sometimes, there might be a narrowing in your bowel caused by a scar from surgery, old inflammation, an intermittent collapse in your bowel or a growth. This can make you feel a build-up of pain and bloating followed by a sudden need to rush to have your bowels open.

4. If there is ulceration or inflammation in your bowel you may have blood or mucus in your stool and you may lose weight.

5. Sometimes you can get pockets in your bowel wall called diverticula. For some people, this causes pain, diarrhoea and a fever.

6. Some people don't have very strong muscle contractions to push the stool along the bowel, so the stool stays in the colon for too long, causing constipation. This is called dysmotility.

7. If there is a narrowing in your rectum, which can be caused by scars from childbirth (having a baby), you can have thin, pencil-like stools, or ribbon-like poo.

8. Sometimes, piles cause bleeding when you wipe, or blood to be mixed in with the stools.

Our easy to navigate tracker enables you to track your food, hydration, mood and poo and to explore how you're feeling, if you're experiencing any symptoms and how much you're moving. This tracker really helps you to understand how your body is working and will give you a great tool to spot patterns, good or bad.

We've even included a gratitude section to help give you little reminder of all the things to be grateful for!

If you do have gut symptoms, you can take your journal to a nutritionist, dietician or GP to help you explain what you're experiencing (we know they'll thank you for it!).

IBS: the story of an irritable gut

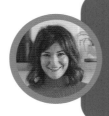

The thing we get asked about most with The Gut Stuff is IBS. It's complex, it's misunderstood and it's definitely on the rise. Every time we have a panel event on this topic, Laura Tilt is at the top of our speed-dial list. Laura is a registered dietitian and health writer and we've never seen a question on IBS she hasn't been able to answer...

Irritable: abnormally sensitive
Bowel: part of the gut, made up of the small bowel (small intestine) and the large bowel (colon and rectum)
Syndrome: a group of symptoms

"The chances are you've heard of irritable bowel syndrome (IBS) or know someone affected by it. IBS is a common digestive condition affecting 1 in 7 adults worldwide. Research shows it's twice as common in women than men (which some scientists think might be related to the impact of female sex hormones on gut function and sensitivity) and is usually diagnosed before the age of 40, although a survey of 2,000 people with IBS conducted by the International Foundation for Gastrointestinal Disorders found that the average amount of time people suffered with symptoms before being diagnosed was 6.6 years.

What exactly is IBS?

IBS is a condition which affects how the gut moves and functions, causing symptoms like pain, bloating, wind and a change in poo habits – typically constipation, diarrhoea or a mixture of both. We can think of the word 'irritable' in IBS as meaning 'abnormally sensitive'. It's a good description for a gut affected by IBS!

What causes IBS?

We still don't know what causes IBS, but there are a few factors that scientists believe play a role. About 60% of people with IBS have super sensitive nerve endings in their gut, which means they are more likely to feel pain and discomfort in response to normal gas production in the large intestine.

There's also evidence that changes in the balance of gut bacteria, stress and previous gut infections can contribute to the development of IBS. And 1 in 3 people with IBS have unusually fast or slow gut motility (movement), which affects how often they poo.

Can IBS be treated?

IBS is a chronic condition – meaning that it persists long-term. This doesn't mean spending the whole time in pain or discomfort though. IBS symptoms fluctuate, and it's possible to go for months or years with symptoms well controlled.

I appreciate that a diagnosis of IBS can sometimes feel like a nothing-y conclusion – something which is diagnosed after everything else has been ruled out – but I want to emphasize that IBS is a very real condition that can significantly impact daily life. I also want to reassure anyone suffering that there are many effective tools that can help improve symptoms.

What can you do if you think you have IBS?

get a medical diagnosis

The first step is to visit your doctor, as IBS shares symptoms with other conditions like coeliac disease, so it's important to get the right diagnosis.

know your IBS

Not all IBS is the same – understanding your symptoms and triggers will help you learn how to manage them. Keeping a food and symptom diary is the first step.

begin with the basics

Eating regular meals, reducing your intake of caffeine, alcohol and spicy foods, and adjusting your fibre consumption are all simple steps that can really make a difference. Learn more at www.bda.uk.com/resource/irritable-bowel-syndrome-diet.html

take stress seriously

Research demonstrates a strong link between stress and IBS severity. Put simply, when you feel stressed, your gut feels it too! Although living completely stress-free isn't possible, learning to manage stress and increase your resilience will help. Gentle exercise, breathing practices and yoga have all been shown to improve symptoms, so it's worth investing time to discover which activities help you to relax and stay calm under pressure.

seek further help

If your symptoms don't improve after trying lifestyle and dietary changes, chat to your doctor about the next steps. In the UK, you can request to see a dietitian who helps with specialist IBS advice. Approaches like CBT (cognitive behavioural therapy), a type of talking therapy which addresses how thoughts affect behaviour, and gut-directed hypnotherapy (which uses guided imagery to help relieve pain) are also available.

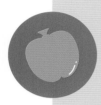

A note on fibre

While most of us can benefit from eating more fibre, if you have an existing gut condition like IBS, increasing fibre may aggravate your symptoms. There isn't enough evidence to say what the right amount of fibre is for people with IBS, so experiment with what you can tolerate and remember that managing your IBS may mean following a different diet to what's recommended for those without a gut condition. As a guide, if you mostly experience loose poos or diarrhoea, choosing lower fibre cereals, reducing fibre from pulses and raw veggies, and avoiding skins, pips and peels can help. If you mostly experience hard small stools (constipation), increasing fibre from oats, wholegrains, linseeds, fruits and vegetables may help. If you are increasing your fibre intake, do so slowly and drink plenty of water too.

FODMAPS: *What are they and what's that got to do with this book? Some types of carbohydrates can go unabsorbed in the small intestine and make it to the large intestine where they get fermented by our microbes. If you have IBS, it can spark the onset of gut symptoms, like gas, pain and change in stools.*

Researchers at Monash University Australia found that by avoiding high FODMAP (Fermentable Oligosaccharides, Disaccharides, Monosaccharides and Polyols) foods – essentially types of carbohydrates – some IBS sufferers had fewer symptoms. Foods high in FODMAPs include starchy foods made from wheat, like bread, pasta and biscuits, specific fruit (like apples), vegetables (onion, garlic and beans) and

certain types of dairy. This resulted in them creating a type of elimination diet, which focuses on avoiding foods high in FODMAPs, which is split into three phases:

1. Elimination,
2. Reintroduction
3. Personalisation.

Not everyone with IBS will benefit from following a low-FODMAP diet and there is no evidence to suggest those without IBS will benefit, plus it also comes with its risks. If you think high FODMAP foods trigger symptoms for you, always consult with a FODMAP dietitian to see if this diet is right for you and to get the support you need. The recipes in this book do not follow a low-FODMAP approach.

orthorexia and the effect on the gut

This next topic is a tricky one and we knew there was only one woman for the job...

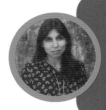

Renee McGregor is a measured, brilliant, sports and eating disorder specialist dietitian with twenty years' experience working in clinical and performance nutrition. When not inspiring others with her incredible work, Renee can be found running in the mountains and chasing the trails, most likely training for a crazy ultra-marathon.

"Orthorexia is an eating disorder defined by 'the obsession with eating correctly or purely'. It has often been associated with the trend to #eatclean. At the time of writing, there is no specific diagnostic criteria due to the complex way it presents in individuals. One of the key difficulties is that so many of the 'wellness' trends of modern life act as a mask to disguise what's really going on. Individuals with orthorexia create strict food and/or exercise rules based on a belief that it will lead to a more healthful life. However, this becomes so obsessive, that any deviation from the rules results in high levels of anxiety, making it impossible for the individual to take part in daily life. As with all eating disorders, in reality, the issue is never food; this is just the medium by which sufferers choose to express their discomfort. In fact, in most

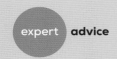
cases, an eating disorder acts as a way to deny and restrict difficult emotions that people do not want to experience. Through their rituals around food and exercise, they aim to contain these difficult emotions, creating an illusion that they are in control and maintaining order.

The food rules created in orthorexia usually result in restricting the body's intake of specific food groups and/or overall energy. This means that there is less energy available to the body for the work it needs to do; when we talk about 'work', we mean the biological processes that go on inside us to keep us alive, as well as any physical activity we do, voluntary and involuntary. When we are in a state of low energy availability, the body will go into preservation mode and down-regulate biological processes, including digestion.

Simply, there is not enough energy for digestion to work efficiently. Transit time through the gut slows, which is known as gastroparesis and the symptoms experienced can often be mistaken for IBS. This is often further exacerbated by the fact that, usually, the individual has a diet very high in fruit and vegetables in order to displace the essential energy they need, which overloads the system further. However, a full history and assessment of the individual should be done, as putting someone who is already restricting their diet on a further restrictive diet, such as the FODMAP (Fermentable Oligo-, Di-, Mono-saccharides and Polyols) diet, can actually make the situation worse as well as feed into their already disordered relationship with food.

If someone is restricting their nutritional intake, this needs to be corrected prior to treating the gut symptoms. Working with a specialist dietitian who can do a full clinical assessment to rule out an underlying restrictive eating disorder as a cause for gut symptoms is critical."

If you think this applies to you or someone you know, speak to your medical professional.

covid and the gut

Naturally Covid-19 and the gut is something we get asked about a lot, so we turned to our wonderful pal and specialist dietitian Sophie Medlin to fill us in on what the research is saying now.

Covid-19 particles are detectable in poo... say whaaaat?

Yep, you heard us right – and what's more, some people still have Covid-19 detectable in their poo for months after they have been infected! Half of those who had contracted the virus still had Covid-19 detectable in their bowel for the week after diagnosis but 4% were still losing viral particles in their poo several months after catching Covid. These inactive viral particles are sometimes called 'coronavirus ghosts' and we think this may be part of the explanation for long-Covid.

The million-dollar question – can Covid-19 cause gut symptoms?

The short answer to this is "yes". As the virus has mutated and changed, we have seen more and more people with gut symptoms due to Covid. For some people these will go away, much like the respiratory aspect of the virus, but for others they may hang around and end up being part of a long-Covid picture.

A study published in March 2022 showed that out of 147 patients with no prior gut issues, 16% reported having persistent gut symptoms around 100 days after they had been hospitalised with Covid-19. Within those who had symptoms, 7.5% had abdominal pain, 6.7% had constipation, 4.1% had diarrhoea and 4.1% had vomiting.

We have also seen that Covid-19 is affecting the gut-brain axis (how our gut and brain communicate), with symptoms such as heartburn, swallowing problems, irritable bowel syndrome (IBS), boating, constipation, and incontinence being reported.

So how exactly does Covid-19 affect the gut?

Get ready for the science-y bit... pop quiz incoming!

There are several possible ways that Covid-19 can cause gut symptoms but we're not currently certain which is the main cause.

What we do know is that the lining of the gut, similar to our lungs and heart, has a large number of cells which are known sites that the spike protein of Covid-19 attaches to, in order to invade our body. These sites are called ACE-2 receptors and within the gut, we have the largest number of them mainly located in the small bowel but also present in the colon, stomach, oesophagus, liver, biliary tract, and pancreas. This means that there are many places in the bowel that Covid-19 can enter the body.

In a healthy gut, ACE-2 has a number of really important roles including helping to regulate blood flow within the gut, protecting the permeability of the bowel wall (keeping some things in and other things out) and optimising muscle contraction which helps with the flow of poo matter through the bowel. They are also involved in preventing inflammatory processes. When the spike protein of Covid-19 attaches to the ACE-2 receptors and invades the cells, they are unable to carry out their normal functions.

Once the virus has entered the intestinal cell walls via the ACE-2 receptors, it can destroy the tight junctions between the cells on the lining of the gut. These vital physical barriers prevent bad bacteria entering our body. Without these working properly, bad bacteria may enter circulation and cause systemic inflammation and infection. It is thought that this contributes to the 'cytokine storm' seen in severe Covid-19 infections.

It is plausible therefore that when Covid-19 has flooded the gut, ACE-2 receptors aren't able to carry out their normal functions which can affect blood flow, the function of the gut lining, the movement or motility within the gut and potentially cause inflammation of the nerves, affecting the gut-brain axis.

And now what we're all wanting to know – how can you treat Covid-19 in the gut?

Unfortunately, we don't yet have any definitive answers as to how we can reverse the gut symptoms from Covid-19. But, based on what we already know here is a roundup of our top tips:

Eating a well-balanced diet (with plenty of plant fibre) will help to support your microbiome in getting back to full health and will also provide your body with lots of vitamins and antioxidants which are important for recovery after any infection.

Glutamine, which is an amino acid, is essential for a healthy gut lining which we know might be compromised during Covid-19 infections. Under physiological stress – such as fighting a virus – our glutamine requirements increase significantly. Some have hypothesised that supplementation with glutamine may help restore the integrity of the gut lining following contraction of Covid-19.

Reducing fermented carbohydrates (FODMAPS) may help to reduce symptoms in those who have ongoing gut problems after catching Covid-19. This should always be done under the supervision of a dietitian as it may cause longer term damage to the gut microbiome if it's not done correctly.

In the case of diarrhoea and constipation, alongside restoring the microbiome through your diet and potentially supplements, using over the counter anti-diarrhoeal or laxative medication may be appropriate. As always, ongoing symptoms need to be seen by your doctor and referral to a dietitian via a self-referral to private clinics is advised.

Lastly, working theories include the use of pre- and probiotics to restore the healthy microbiome we require to dampen down inflammation and support healthy digestion. Researchers are looking at the potential benefits of pre- and probiotics in the prevention of severe Covid-19 but there isn't any clear evidence to show what the best strains would be at the moment.

Still with us? Delve deeper...

What is the role of the microbiome?

In mouse studies, rodents without a healthy microbiome produce far more ACE-2 expression across the bowel than those with a healthy microbiome. This creates more sites for Covid-19 to attach to, which may increase the level of infection within the gut and how long the symptoms last for.

Covid-19 infection disrupts gut bacteria by decreasing the proportions of probiotic (good) bacteria and increasing the numbers of pathogenic (bad) bacteria. This may contribute to the bowel symptoms people are experiencing post Covid-19 infection as Covid will have reduced their numbers of good bacteria.

We also know that people who take anti-acid medication (PPIs), often had worse outcomes from Covid-19. This is thought to be due to the negative impact of PPIs on our gut bacteria.

It is likely that having a healthy microbiome (gut bacteria) may offer a better physical barrier throughout the gut, making it harder for the Covid-19 virus to find and adhere to ACE-2 receptors.

We also think that the short-chain fatty acids produced by beneficial bacteria within the gut and the respiratory tract are highly protective against a severe Covid-19 infection. They are shown to promote anti-Covid-19 antibody production and therefore prevent the development of a Covid-19 infection at a cellular level. Short-chain fatty acids from bacteria also have a strong anti-inflammatory effect which is thought to protect from the 'cytokine storm'.

It may seem obvious, given the information above to say that people with low microbial diversity or a poor microbiome are more likely to have worse outcomes if they do come into contact with Covid-19 and this is a very reasonable hypothesis, but we don't have definitive proof of this as yet.

bullsh*t bin (sorry mum)

And now we're on to the *how*. As we're walking out of the school playground and back home to digest all the science we've learned, have a wee walk past our new bin, it's like the official charts top rundown of all the nutrition nonsense we see and hear. So, turn the radio up and tune in to the bullsh*t bin!

Skinny teas

These are teas (yes, teabags!) that claim to make you lose weight but are really just expensive flavoured water. Some contain caffeine, a diuretic, and senna, a laxative – weeing and pooing more may make you feel lighter but these ingredients can cause other issues and come with side effects like bloating, cramps and diarrhoea. Long-term use of senna can also impair how well your gut works, meaning you become dependent on it to make you go. Not cool. Not cool at all.

Cleanses, detoxes, lemon water and celery juice

Aside from lemon potentially eroding the enamel from your teeth, there is no evidence that foods or drinks detox your body – your body is detoxifying all the time. Providing you have a working gut, kidneys and liver, your body has all it needs to detox.

'Superfoods'

We think most foods have the power to be 'superfoods'. Whether they provide you with gut-loving fibre or polyphenols (see page 126), or the taste of a cinnamon bun takes you back to being a carefree 10-year-old, the physical and mental benefits food can provide means there are no true superfoods. Save your cash, avoid expensive powders and exotic ingredients and instead eat as many plant foods (and colours) as possible and you won't go far wrong.

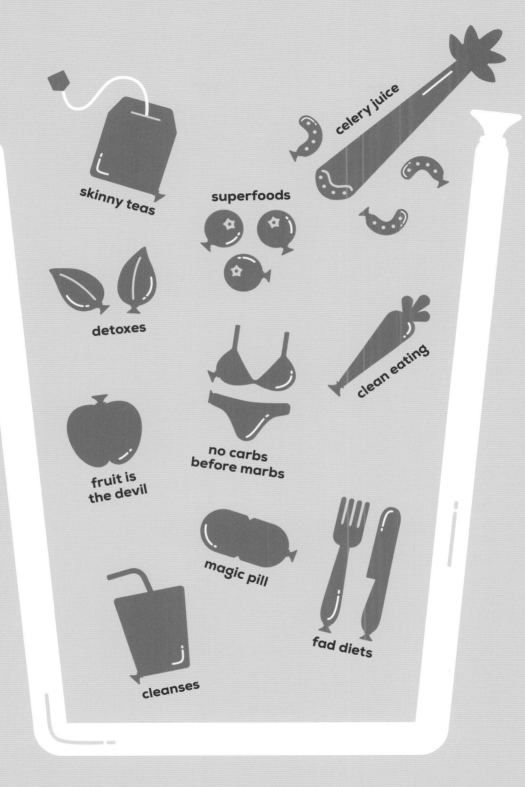

Clean eating

We hope the fad of #cleaneating passes. A gut-loving diet is one that contains an abundance of plant foods, but that doesn't mean you can't enjoy other ingredients that bring you pleasure as part of a balanced diet. Clean eating has also seen the rise of disordered eating, which has very serious consequences on your gut indeed.

"No carbs before Marbs"

If you want to starve your hardworking microbes of fuel to do their thing, don't starve them of carbs. Wholegrains in particular are a really important source of fibre to fuel your microbes, so if you suddenly cut them out, you are going to negatively affect your gut microbes.

Fad diets

They are called fads for a reason. Do your research and speak to a professional if you want to change your diet.

Magic pill

No matter how many supplements you pop, there is no magic pill for a happy gut. We are all individual, as are our guts.

"Fruit is the Devil"

Fruit gets a bad rap and it shouldn't. Fruit contains important fibre, nutrients and polyphenols for your gut. Try to have it in its whole form, rather than juiced, to get maximum benefits.

The bottom line

Food provides not only nourishment but also enjoyment. Be informed and make educated decisions (that means not treating social media like an encyclopaedia of wellness) when thinking about your gut. If common sense tells you it's too good to be true that's because it is!

myth-busting
toolkit

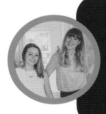

After reading their book *Is Butter a Carb?*, we knew exactly the two gals to arm you with your Inspector-Gadget-style myth-busting toolkit to detect all the nutri-nonsense crimes out there. Enter Helen West and Rosie Saunt of The Rooted Project (slow-mo Charlie's-Angels-style walk)...

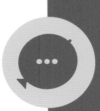

"Nutrition myths are everywhere. From claims about the toxicity of whole food groups (e.g. carbs kill!) to the reductive focus on individual nutrients as a cure-all, nutrition myths are used to sell us a vast array of food products, diets and lifestyles, often with flashy advertising and strong, clear-cut messages. On the surface, these messages are appealing. They simplify the complex area of diet and health and neatly commodify it into something we can purchase and control. Got cancer? Take these vitamins. Feel tired? Follow this detox. Want abs? Buy these appetite suppressants. You get the picture. Bold nutrition claims speak to our (very human) desire for simplicity, they draw on our anxieties about our bodies and health and sell us straightforward solutions and quick fixes. Even knowing this, there are so many people out there exploiting the knowledge gaps and uncertainties in this complex field, that sorting the truths from the half-truths and downright nutri-nonsense can feel like a dizzying task. But you don't need to be an expert in nutrition to navigate the myths. There's often some telltale signs that a claim or product may not be quite as it seems.

So, here are our **top ten** tips for spotting nutrition nonsense:

① A focus on single foods or nutrients
Bold or scary claims about single foods or nutrients causing disease are a sign you should be wary. Health is complex, so these claims are likely to be untrue or, at the very least, overblown.

② Offers a simple fix for a complex problem
If something sounds too good to be true (e.g. it is offering a single, simple solution, like a vitamin pill, for a complex health problem), then it probably is.

③ Uses 'hot bodies' or celebs to bolster claims
"Eat like me, look like me" is a common unspoken marketing trick for many food products. Are they linking their product with a look? Or claiming a food changes your appearance?

④ Proof via anecdotes
People's experiences and stories are valid and important, but we can't use them as 'proof' that something will work in the same way for us.

⑤ Promotes one way to eat as the right way
Have they come up with THE way to eat for good health? Healthy eating can be reached in many different ways, so if they are promoting their diet as the one and only road to 'healthy', be critical.

⑥ Is it selling you a 'detox'?
Are they promoting the idea that our environment is toxic and that we need specific products to detox our bodies? Eating well supports good health, but special products aren't needed to improve our body's capacity to detox itself.

7   A focus on 'natural' as best

Saying something is 'natural' makes it sound like it is wholesome or pure and, most importantly, 'safe'. It's comforting and appealing. But 'natural' isn't synonymous with any of these things. Many dangerous things are 'natural' – like cyanide.

8   Is it actually an advert?

Check that the article you are reading is actually an article. Paid promotions for nutrition products like diets or supplements can be dressed up as impartial communications.

9   Promotes a diet as the sole alternative to proven medical therapies

Any products or services which advise that you should reject and avoid your doctor in favour of their services should be treated with caution.

10   Uses sensationalist language like 'toxic' or 'poisonous'

If a communication is sensationalist and using language that invokes fear, then view claims with scepticism."

You're now ready. Go, go gadgets GO.

live that
gut life

chapter 2

top trio of gut-loving principles

As we touched upon before, unfortunately there isn't a magic ingredient for good gut health... we've asked scientists, doctors, dietitians and nutritionists and the three simple tips that come up time and time again are...

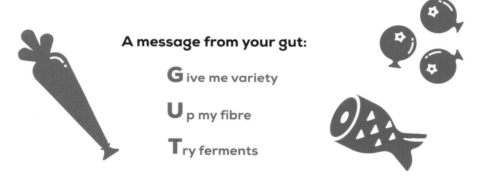

A message from your gut:

Give me variety

Up my fibre

Try ferments

If you keep all the different microbes happy, they can do incredible things like help to control your blood sugar, produce vitamins, manage cholesterol and hormonal balance, prevent you from getting infections, control the calories that you absorb and store, communicate with your nervous system and brain, influence your bone strength and so much more. Therefore, for each recipe later in the book, we've supplied a key (see page 131) so you can keep track of all the variety, fibre and ferments in every meal, which leads us very nicely on to the next section of gut tips...

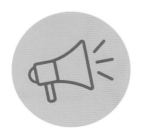

Providing you've not been medically advised otherwise, we want you to ditch the restriction and diet mentality and think about what you can ADD for your gut, not take away.

the GUT tips

Variety – the spice of gut life

OK, what does the science say? Well, a study found that people who ate thirty-plus different plant-based foods a week were found to have a more diverse mix of gut microbes than those who ate less than ten. Think about thirty different types of music lovers at the festival; the more bands (plant-based foods) there are, the more people will be enjoying the festival as everyone will have something they like! Thirty plants a week may seem like a high number to hit but the recipes in this book have 'gut' you covered.

7 ways to up your variety

1 Tuning in to what you eat can help you spot patterns and see how much variety you are really getting. Note down what you've eaten and tally up the number of different plants you've consumed over the week. Did you make it to thirty?

2 Research shows that if we plan meals ahead and use shopping lists, we are more likely to eat more vegetables and healthier meals. Set aside 30 minutes at the end of the week to plan the week ahead or keep a notepad to jot down your shopping needs. We've listed all our go-to ingredients in this book (see pages 106–113).

3 Use mixed bags of salad as they usually contain over three different types of leaves – win!

4 Use all the colours of peppers (each counts separately!) – different colours mean more points and points mean prizes!

5 Buy a bag of mixed frozen veg – the freezer is your friend.

6 Make your own nut and seed mixes to sprinkle on salads or soups for a bit of crunch. You can get up to five or six cheeky points here! (See recipe on page 229).

7 Switch up your pasta and include lentil, pea and chickpea pasta with your favourite sauce (yes, really!).

Fibre

Fibre is the unsung hero of nutrition, like the bassist in the band whose name nobody knows. Adults need 30g (1 oz) of fibre a day, but 90% of us simply aren't getting enough. Like adults, children in the UK aren't eating enough either – the amount children need varies by age (2–3 years = 15g/½ oz; 5–11 years = 20g/¾ oz; 11–16 = 25g/1 oz). With the increased consumption of processed foods, lack of fruit and vegetables in our diets and popularity of low-carbohydrate diets and/or fasting, fibre has been somewhat cast aside and we're here to bring it BACK.

Great, so we've got to up it, but where do we get it? Getting fibre from vegetables and fruit alone is tricky, so you need whole grains, nuts and seeds and pulses to add to the mix. Also, do your gut bugs a favour and don't cut carbs. This is where our easy peasy recipes come in; each meal being high in fibre (at least 6g per 100g fibre in each portion).

You may have heard of soluble and insoluble fibres but we now know (thanks science) that there are many different types of fibre and it's this variety that's the key. Your microbes each enjoy different foods and so focusing on just one type of food (even a 'superfood') won't give you the gut benefits of eating a variety of different plants.

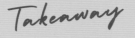

What is fibre?
The non-digestible carbohydrates found in plants that we can't digest but our gut microbes can.

Where can you get it?
It's either naturally found in plants that we ingest or fibres can also be isolated or manufactured and added to foods.

7 ways to up your fibre

1   Don't let veg and fruit skins go to waste, just give them a good scrub. Grate carrots with the skin on, roast potatoes without peeling (we promise they're just as crispy) and save yourself a load of mess by keeping the skin on beetroot.

2   Go for wholegrain over refined white versions of the same food. Try and swap white rice, pasta and bread for wholegrain varieties.

3   Add nuts and/or seeds to breakfasts, soups, salads or stir-fries, or snack on them with a piece of fruit. We've always got a bag of nuts in our handbag or a jar in the house for snacking during the day.

4   Understand what's on a label: 6g or more per 100g = high fibre, 3–5.9g per 100g = source of fibre.

5   Add beans, like butter beans or chickpeas or lentils to meals, like adding red lentils to Bolognese sauce (see page 176). These are great to bulk out and add extra nutrients to soups, stews and salads.

6   Start the day right. Enjoy oats or bran for breakfast and you avoid all those ultra-processed, sugar-laden cereals.

7   Get to know your numbers – check out our fibre table to see which foods give you the most fibre for your buck. We think you'll be surprised how much fibre is in certain foods – we know we were!

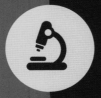

The plant wall contains around 95% of all fibre (need a reason to keep the skins on your tatties?) and the type of plant and the part (root, leaf or stem) you are eating will make a difference to the type of fibre and quantity it contains.

Ferments:
the tangtastic addition

Fermented foods have been around since Neolithic times. They're often associated with a hefty price tag, making them something a lot of us wouldn't even think to put in our shopping baskets. However, they don't need to be expensive and, once you've learned the basic principles, you can make fermented foods really easily at home (see pages 248–269). If done right (this is key!), fermented food can be a great source of bacteria and their by-products.

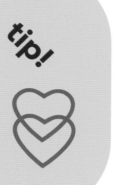

A note about shop-bought ferments: always check that they contain live bacteria and aren't pasteurized or that they contain 'live cultures' (often added back in after pasteurization), otherwise you may lose the potential benefits that the community of microbes bring.

Why ferment food?

Historically, food was fermented to simply make it last longer and preserve it for consumption later (often by just making a brine with salt). Due to the bacteria and yeasts, fermented food is also tasty and may, in some ferments, increase the food's nutritional value. When bacteria and yeasts ferment food, they produce something called metabolites. These metabolites include lactic acid, vitamins and exopolysaccharides (sugar molecules) and may support our health and wellbeing (we are still trying to understand how and why).

Lots of different foods can be fermented, such as dairy, fish (yes really!), vegetables, cereals and fruits. The key bacteria found in fermented foods include Lactococcus, Lactobacillus, Streptococcus and Leuconostoc but yeasts and other bacteria also feature, depending on the ferment. The number of microbes (and their by-products) present will depend on how and where the ferment is made, how it's stored and what it's made from.

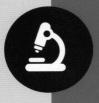

Different ferments will contain different bacteria, cultures and by-products (variety is also key when it comes to ferments; two principles in one!). We're going to be speed-dating different types of ferments later, then showing you how to make your own to add into all our recipes.

The sourdough bakers in San Francisco say their bread has a unique taste because of the unique microbes that inhabit their mothers (the sourdough starter kind).

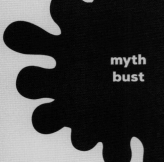

myth bust

Why do some ferments say 'probiotic' on the packet? Well, 'pro' means 'life' in Greek, so when food contains live bacteria, cultures and/or yeasts it is often termed a probiotic. However, you are not legally allowed to call a food a probiotic in the UK so you may see 'live cultures' instead. And don't get ferments confused with pickles (like we did!) – they are a totally different thing.

fermented foods:
is there evidence?

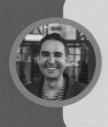

Miguel Toribio-Mateas is a clinical neuroscientist by day and (like us) a DJ by night. He's the wackiest scientist we know (in the most brilliant way!) and has a wicked sense of humour, plus an extensive background in nutrition practice and research. As part of his visiting research fellowship in microbiome and mental health at the School of Applied Sciences, London South Bank University, he studied fermented foods, so is PERFECT to tackle this subject...

"Conducting research on any kind of food, especially temperamental live foods, can be tricky because of the amount of confounders (other factors that can affect the result). Imagine taking part in a study on the effects of 'food X' on any particular symptom, let's say bloating. A researcher would also need to be aware of other factors including:

- The effects of how hydrated you were during the study, or whether you smoked or drank alcohol.

- The effect of how well and how long you slept.

- Your physical activity level/exercise.

- Ultimately, was food X definitively responsible for the change in your symptoms? And what potential weight did other foods you ate alongside food X carry?

Next, comes the complication with what I am measuring. When it comes to gut health and its effect on the health of the rest of your body (physical and mental), it is difficult to find one indicator as an absolute marker of health. Clinicians use these indicators (called biomarkers) when diagnosing a condition. One such example is calprotectin, a molecule produced by immune cells in the gut – high levels are found in people with inflammatory bowel disease (IBD), Crohn's disease or ulcerative colitis. Another issue is how the results are collected. Self-reported symptoms are often reported using a questionnaire to help the researcher understand the severity of the patient's bloating, cramping and discomfort. But as symptoms are experienced differently by different individuals, this is a very subjective measure and so not necessarily the most reliable.

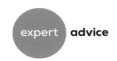

When researchers run drug clinical trials, there's a typical series of phases the drugs have to pass through before and after they are approved so that they can be prescribed and marketed for a specific use. This process isn't relevant for most food products, but fermented foods are a little different. Why, you may be asking? Well, fermented foods like kefir, sauerkraut, kimchi, miso, kombucha, etc. have been used traditionally in different cultures for centuries, but now researchers want to assess their value as foods with a specific function (beyond nutrients), or as 'functional foods'. If these functions are backed by research and approved by the relevant authorities, it means health claims about their therapeutic or medicinal properties can be made about a specific fermented food. Without rigorous research, you cannot make such claims. So even if clinical research on food is always going to be a little 'funky', it is still very much needed.

In my research role as Lead Neuroscientist at the Bowels and Brains Lab at London South Bank University, I've been assessing what kefir, sauerkraut, kimchi and fermented vegetable juice do to the gut and also to the brain. To figure out the effects of these foods on the gut, researchers have looked at changes in the type and amount of bacteria, such as Lactobacilli and Bifidobacteria. For the brain, we've used psychometric tests to look at how the brain changes (or not) in response to these types of foods. These two types of results (the effect on gut microbes and the brain) are then fed into a statistical analysis phase to identify patterns between the food and changes to gut symptoms, such as bloating or stool consistency, but also to mood, attention/focus or memory.

Trials cost a lot of money (sometimes millions) and can take a long time to complete, which means thousands of man/woman hours and a lot of stress in the lab, chasing participants, analyzing the data and writing up the results, aiming to get them published after an exhausting peer review. (What's a peer review? To be published in a reputable paper, a research study must be peer reviewed – this means it gets looked over by other researchers to validate the study for publication. It is a form of self-regulation and ensures a high standard in the publication of research studies.)

Despite all of these hurdles, this is an enormously exciting time to be involved in clinical research on the effects of fermented foods on health, and it feels hugely enriching to be able to contribute to people's health by providing them with scientific evidence on how foods we've been eating for centuries work by interacting with their gut bugs."

supercharge your store cupboards

Knowing how to stock your kitchen – from cupboards to freezer – makes it so much easier to include more gut-loving (and tasty!) foods in your diet. In this section, we'll walk you through the best ways to maximize the potential in your kitchen, with our top ingredients to keep on-hand and help you live that gut life.

larder

Having a good sort out of your larder and streamlining what you store, not only helps you keep track of what you have but if you can see what's in stock, you are more likely to use it. This doesn't have to be expensive or require a foraging trip to find exotic ingredients.

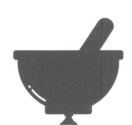

1 **Herbs and spices** – all add variety for your gut microbes.
Turmeric – great for adding colour and an earthy flavour to curries.
Cinnamon – add to smoothies, stewed fruits, banana bread and porridge for a warming feel.
Smoked paprika – great for Mexican or Spanish flavours; we like ours in baked eggs and on sweet potato fries and hummus.
Oregano – gives instant Mediterranean flavour; mix it into salad dressings or use on roast veg.
Chilli flakes – we love chilli on our hummus or to take a dish up a notch.
Ground ginger – add to curries and stir-fries for extra flavour, and no grating needed!
Garlic powder – saves the faff of crushing it (and no smelly hands!).

2 **Dry goods** – a few staples help to increase variety in your meals.
Dried pulses – our favourites are beans, peas, chickpeas and lentils – a little goes a long way, but you'll need to soak them in water overnight.
Quinoa – pronounce it however you like!
Wholegrain pasta, lentil pasta and chickpea pasta – great alternatives to regular pasta.
Soba noodles – we love these in ramen; great at soaking up broth.
Wholegrain couscous – makes a super speedy lunch.
Pearl barley – good to add to soups or to use instead of other grains.
Oats – for making overnight oats, flapjacks, porridge or savoury oats.
Nuts and seeds – buy mixed bags to get those variety numbers up.
Nutritional yeast – sounds random but a great cheese substitute! If you're vegan, look for added vitamin B12.

3 **Cans** – great for convenience and boosting nutritional value of meals.
Chopped tomatoes and coconut milk – for quick sauces and curries.
Beans and pulses – mixed ones will up those variety points.

4 **Oil and vinegar**
Good-quality extra virgin olive oil – packed full of polyphenols.
Apple cider vinegar – with the mother.
Tahini – great for dressings and hummus.
Tamari – for depth of flavour.

fridge

Having a system for your fridge and freezer can make it a lot easier to use and if you can see what you've stored, it will encourage you to use. We use glass jars (and recycle the ones food came in) and glass boxes to help us see what we've got.

1 **Top shelf** – stuff you've made.
Stewed fruits – we try whatever we can find.
Pre-cooked vegetables – always do a bit extra at dinner for the next day.
Pesto – we use whatever nuts we have to hand and then something green – basil, spinach or rocket.
Hummus – homemade or store-bought.

2 **Middle shelf** – dairy and fermented foods.
Artisan cheese – these are the ones that typically contain plenty of bacteria (if unpasteurised).
Live yogurt – always read the label – look for 'live cultures' or 'live bacteria'.
Kefir – milk or water (see pages 264–265).
Kombucha – make your own (see page 266).
Ferments – we try cabbage or root veg, or make your own (see pages 248–269).

3 **Bottom shelf**
Meats
Fish

4 **Vegetable / salad / fruit drawer** – aim for as much variety and as many colours as possible.

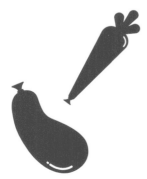

freezer

Frozen food shouldn't be shunned – it's a great way of having nourishing food at hand, avoiding food waste and making cooking cheaper and more efficient. These are our freezer staples to help get variety:

① Fruit and veg

Fruit – berries of any kind, diced apple, sliced banana, avocado, mango, pineapple, pomegranate, rhubarb. Top on porridge, add to kefir (not the water kind) or have as a snack.

Vegetables – spinach, mixed veg, peas, sweetcorn, mixed peppers, green beans, mushrooms – the list goes on! Just throw a few handfuls into your hot meals for an extra dose of goodness – perfect for curries, pastas, stir-fries and stews.

Roasted or grilled veg/ratatouille mix – perfect for last-minute meals – top with fish, lentils or make a pasta sauce.

Ready-chopped onions and garlic – super-easy to add to the base of most dishes to increase fibre and variety and save on time when you're busy during the week.

Herbs – chop and freeze in little pouches; ready to go. This was a game changer for us!

② Quick snacks

Muffins and energy balls – freeze separately – that way you just lift out what you need.

Vegetable and fruit lolly pops – made using a mix of both and kefir or live yogurt.

Pre-sliced sourdough – super easy to toast a slice or two when you need (and prevents waste!).

③ Batch cooking

Sauces and bases – we freeze portions of homemade pasta sauce in large ice cube trays so it is super easy to lift out.

Meals – you can batch cook all sorts of meals like curries, soups, lasagne, fish pie, bean burgers and even banana pancakes for quick access on busier days – the freezer is your friend!

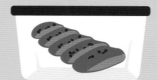

what: *chilli*
when: *17.09.23*
portion: *two*

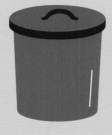

sort it, so you don't
have to chuck it

use clear containers

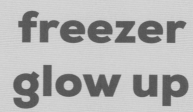

freeze in
portion sizes

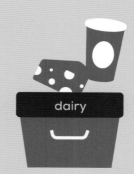

freezer
glow up

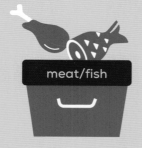

meat/fish

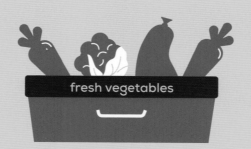

fresh vegetables

dairy

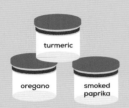

herbs
& spices

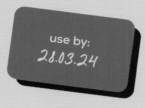

use by

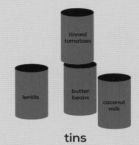

tins

food cupboard glow up

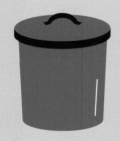

sort it, so you don't
have to chuck it

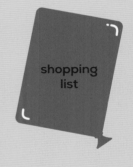

shopping
list

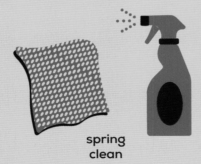

spring
clean

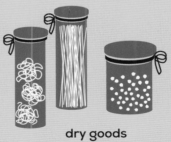

dry goods

simple swaps

Our aim has always been to make gut health accessible for everyone, which is why we've got some simple swaps for you to implement a bit at a time to help you on your gut health journey. Take it steady and keep it simple – you don't have to go from zero to hero as soon as you put this book down.

Still a bit confused? Pick one of these simple swaps to start with...

Swap white for brown

- Change white pasta for wholegrain – white pasta (2g fibre) vs wholegrain (7.5g fibre).

- Instead of white rice, try brown, red or black rice – white rice (1g fibre) vs brown (4g fibre).

- Swap low-fibre cereal for a fibre-dense variety, such as bran or oat-based cereals cornflakes (0.8g fibre) vs bran flakes (5.4g fibre).

- Try wholegrain sourdough or rye bread, slice of white bread (1g fibre) vs slice of seeded wholegrain (5g fibre).

If you aren't a fan of wholegrain versions of your white favourites, try introducing them into your diet slowly (e.g. use half white/half brown rice) until you get used to the different texture and flavour. Making this simple switch will help you reach 30g fibre a day.

Vegetable boxes

Instead of opting for your usual online food shop, why don't you give a veg box a whirl? Vegetable and fruit boxes often work out to be great value for good-quality produce and a lot of the schemes support local farms. It's also another way of trying to get more plant-based variety over the course of the week as the contents change regularly depending on what's in season. There are lots of great options out there, from odd-shaped veg to farm-to-home boxes. It's a great way of getting near thirty different plant-based foods a week to support that diverse ecosystem in your gut.

Make the freezer your friend!

You tend to get more food for your money by buying frozen and you won't be compromising on quality. Spinach, berries and mixed veg are great freezer staples and give you the opportunity to increase variety without food waste.

Swap regular pasta...

...for chickpea, lentil or pea pasta to increase the different plant-based foods in your diet.

Yogurt

Where a recipe calls for yogurt, replace with live natural yogurt or kefir.

Chocolate

Swap milk chocolate for dark (anything north of 75% cocoa solids) to increase your consumption of gut-loving polyphenols.

Roasted veg

Swap skinless roasted veg for skin on where you can; just be sure to give your veg a good scrub.

Condiments

If you are a condiment lover, swap your usual condiments for sauerkraut or kimchi. You'll be amazed how your taste buds change to crave their fermented flavours.

Soup

Swap your cuppa soup for miso soup.

Fizzy pop

Swap for kombucha or, if that's going too far, sparkling water with some fresh herbs or mint to reduce your intake of artificial preservatives and sweeteners.

Ditch the guilt!

Enjoy your food. Digestion starts before food passes your lips – enjoying and looking forward to the food you eat is just as important as chewing properly. If you are holding your nose and downing a celery juice, you aren't going to digest it properly.

it ain't just about food

Sometimes it is about more than just WHAT we eat. As we said, we've got your back. Our top tips to support your gut mean making use of the bullsh*t bin (see pages 90–92) and focusing on a few simple things...

We have so many tools in our armoury – by using the gnashers we were made with, adding a pinch of consistency, plus a dash of mindfulness, we should have the perfect potion to set up some gut days ahead...

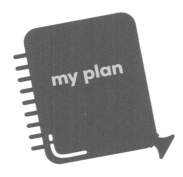

my plan

the science of habit forming

It is all well and good knowing what to eat but how do you put that into practice? How many times have you said you're going to take up a new habit only for it to last a week? Both hands up for us!

Before we delve into the HOW, let's explain the WHAT.

A habit is a behaviour that you repeat regularly – it could be an action (like planning your meals or writing a diary), a routine (like shopping on a Sunday) or a lifestyle (like making sure you're active). Eventually, these behaviour patterns become subconscious and part of your day-to-day life – this is great news if the habit is a positive one, and even better if it's going to support you living that gut life!

Takin' the easy way outtt...

When given the choice, us humans often pick the easiest, quickest or most enjoyable option (we know that's the case for us!). Now, there's nothing wrong with this but when it comes to choosing an action that supports your gut, creating simple habits that become part of your routine may be better than the perceived easiest option. For example, if you always find yourself not knowing what to cook and reaching for the simplest and quickest option (like a ready meal or takeaway), planning your meals ahead and making a weekly habit of it may help you to eat a more gut-friendly diet.

The formation of a habit isn't as complex as you might think, but there are steps (and a little effort) required up front to make that habit stick. For an action to become a habit, it needs to be repeated and is often triggered by a cue (e.g. washing your hands after going to the loo).

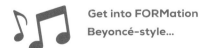 Get into FORMation Beyoncé-style...

Gotcha. OK, gimme the HOW.

- Decide on what goal you want to achieve (we've got some ideas for you below).

- Choose a simple action that you will do at a set time (e.g. making breakfast the night before).

- Plan when and where you will do this (e.g. 7 p.m. when cooking dinner in the kitchen) and your cue (e.g. planner on the fridge).

- Do the action (e.g. making breakfast).

- Keep doing it at the same time. You might find it useful to keep track of it by writing it down in a diary – you may find our gut diary helpful here (available from our website).

- Once it becomes second nature = habit formed.

Great... so a couple of days and I'm all set?

Not quite. You may have heard that it takes twenty-one days to form a habit – we love facts and figures but the truth is, it depends on the habit you're trying to implement, who you are and a lot of other circumstances. One piece of research looked at how long it took adults to form healthy habits, from dietary changes to physical activity – on average, it took sixty-six days but there was quite a range, from 18–254 days! So keep that in mind.

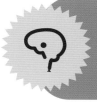 It's also important to remember that you won't derail your efforts by not doing it every day (a common misconception).

Here is a little platter of 'gut' habits to pick from...

One more plant

Plant-based variety is so important when it comes to gut health. Assess each meal you make and ask yourself: Is there one more plant I could add? It could be herbs, seeds or a different kind of vegetable. The cue is looking at your plate or ticking off your plant count in a diary or on a tally-mark table on the fridge. We can help you with that... our handy variety checklist magnet allows you to keep track of variety in your shopping list and help you reach thirty different plants a week.

Plan the meals you make at home in advance

Choose the same day each week to sit down and do this and stick a reminder on your fridge (or use our meal planner magnet).

Sit down to eat (and don't pick while making food)

Put away your phone, chew properly and be ready to digest. This is one of the easiest and most underrated things you can do, and it's free! Cues: If you're standing, don't eat.

Make your own fermented food

Start slow, set time aside once a month to make your ferment or sourdough. Cues: Put your ferment schedule somewhere visible, regularly check on your ferment, care for it like a pet and, when it's done, have it in sight in your fridge so you remember to add it to dishes. There are loads of ferments coming up later, see pages 248–269.

Fibre-fuelled breakfast

Make your breakfast the night before so it's ready to grab and go. Our overnight oats (see pages 136–139) are super simple and we have lots of toppings to tickle your fancy.

Use a diary

If you're experiencing gut symptoms, try a notebook or diary to record what you're eating and the symptoms you're experiencing. This will help you tune in to your body and spot patterns that might be helpful.

chew, chew and chew again

We know this sounds EMBARRASSINGLY SIMPLE but, "Do you chew enough?" As we learnt back in biology class (see page 16), digestion doesn't begin in your stomach; it begins before you even put food in your mouth. We've all experienced the mouthwatering sensation when it's just our eyeballs having the feast, and this is enough to kick off the digestive process. It's natural that we're all busy and guilty of ramming a sandwich down our necks as we hot-foot it across the city. But even though everyone else in your train carriage knows about your tuna roll, your gut doesn't, and we need to warn it... "Ready the troops, tastiness incoming!"

You should be trying to chew your food 20–30 times (we know, seems a lot!) before you swallow to make sure it is properly broken down to make less work for the rest of the orchestra waiting below (see pages 16–21).

Some smart Alec/a*se once asked us, "What about soup?" – don't be that guy... use your judgement with soup!

We're naturally food hoovers, so we've started using mini sand-timers to train ourselves not to finish our meal until the last grain of sand has dropped – very *Crystal Maze* and a good game for kids too.

mindful eating

So, some of the time it's not about WHAT we eat but HOW we eat. For this we'd like you to imagine you're on a date... with yourself.

- Look forward to your food as you would a hot date. Don't eat foods because they are 'good' for you but because they are nourishing, and you enjoy them – kinda like picking a dating partner.

- You should always focus on the person you're dining with, so sit down to eat and prepare for digestion. Turn off distractions and focus on your meal/date.

- Rest your knife and fork between mouthfuls and chew your food. Savour the flavours before swallowing. Imagine you're having a conversation and having to leave gaps to chat/boast/giggle/run for the hills. As for date chat suggestions, here's a little starter for 10 to ask yourself before/during eating:

  ○ Are you responding to an emotional want, thirst or your body's needs?

  ○ Is your stomach gurgling? Do you feel hungry or do your energy levels feel low?

  ○ Are you reaching for food due to a stressful event?

  ○ Have your food choices been impacted by your emotions? Could you eat nourishing foods to support how you feel instead?

  ○ Are you focused on your food or is your mind distracted?

  ○ How does your food taste, smell and feel?

  ○ Are you full? Check in with yourself during your meal.

to fast or not to fast?

—

You've probably heard a lot about fasting, 5:2, 12-hour, 16:8. But what is best for your gut microbes? The truth is, we don't really know, and it varies greatly from person to person, depending on your health and stage of life. Some research shows that giving your gut a break overnight can help your gut microbes to flourish, but whether whole days of food restriction benefits them, regardless of any other purported benefits, the jury is out. Do what you find works for you but pay attention to your body and no one else's... you do you.

could having a good social circle improve our gut health?

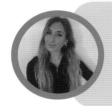

Like eating with friends? We asked nutritionist Annabel Sparrow, who also has a degree in psychology, to look at the evidence on the theory that eating together may actually be better for our guts.

More and more research is highlighting that having strong social connections positively impacts our mental health. But did you know it could also improve your gut health?

If you've read any of our other articles, you'll know our gut microbiome is a powerhouse of positive health outcomes, from balancing our blood sugar to managing hormones and even impacting our mental health through our gut brain axis (along with much more!).

Therefore, it may not come as a big surprise that new research indicates that socialising may be linked to a healthy and diverse gut microbiota.

A recent study analysed social behaviour and the gut microbiome in a community of wild chimps. Researchers found higher social interaction led to increased levels of 'good' gut bacteria. What's more, the microbiome composition was similar across the group – sharing is caring after all.

Why is this happening? The researchers suggest this may be because through increased socialising, there are more opportunities for bacteria to transmit and thus diversify, as well as potentially reducing stress levels. Both of which could result in a healthier gut microbiome.

We know, you're not an animal, why does this matter to you? Well, the evidence doesn't stop there, in fact this is further supported by emerging research in humans. A longitudinal study of nearly 60 years, found socialness in family and friends was associated with differences in microbiota. Positively, married individuals with close sustained relationships had a more diverse gut microbiota.

The science doesn't stop there. Two further human studies found having a larger social network and higher levels of social support and social engagement is correlated with greater diversity within the gut microbiome.

All of this suggests that socialising and spending more time with your friends and family may play a role in promoting gut health and the diversity of your gut microbiome. Music to our ears!

This really is just the beginning of research in this area. Further research on larger and more diverse human populations is needed to confirm findings and make them generalisable.

However, this emerging research does suggest getting friendly could be making not just you happy but your gut happy too. Plus, it supports spending more time with your loved ones, which, let's face it, can never be a bad thing.

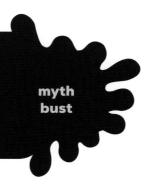

'Don't drink liquids with food' is a myth. There's no robust evidence to support this or to say that liquids impair the digestion of food. There's some research that alcohol and caffeine may have an effect but it depends on the type and quantity.

myth bust

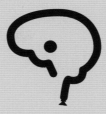

Living, working or even just eating alone can mean we fall into habits that aren't doing our guts any favours (think slumped in front of the TV, mindlessly chowing down). Having the radio or a podcast on can bring a feeling of company while still allowing you to focus on your date with your gut.

alcohol

Excess alcohol can aggravate your gut, from affecting how well you digest your food to making things move a bit quicker than usual! Too much alcohol can inhibit the digestive enzymes you produce, which means your food won't be digested and absorbed as well as it could be.

Undigested food makes more work for your gut bacteria and when your bacteria has to work harder, you produce more gas – cue bloating and windiness when you've had a few too many bevvies. There's a lovely bacteria that lives in the mucus lining of your gut – remember *Akkermansia* from the job description on page 25? When you drink a lot of alcohol, the mucus lining can get damaged and this can reduce the amount of *Akkermansia* as well as other important microbes.

There's only one man we could draft in to answer our many, many questions on alcohol (usually via WhatsApp on hungover Sundays: "How much? What kind? Why is this hangover so bloomin' awful?").

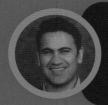

Gautam Mehta is a liver specialist and honorary consultant at University College London, with many incredible research projects on the go, but he took a break to answer these (very important!) questions for us all...

Is red wine REALLY good for you?

"Research shows there is an association between moderate red wine consumption (see opposite for what 'moderation' means) and increased diversity of gut microbiota, which in turn has been associated with a healthier gut and possible benefits for cardiovascular and other metabolic diseases. Before you grab a bottle of red, the key word in this last sentence is 'association' – this doesn't prove cause and effect. The study in question looked at a snapshot of the gut microbiome and compared this with alcohol and dietary information in the study population, rather than conducting a prospective intervention study with a control group. To me and you, that means people self-reported consumption and diet instead of being prescribed a diet and specific units of alcohol to drink (and people tend to underreport on these things). Your microbiome has the ability to change very quickly, so a one-off stool sample doesn't always give a clear picture. Nevertheless, the effect seen was much greater for red wine than for white wine or other alcoholic drinks, which may be because of the greater concentration of polyphenols in red wine. Polyphenols seem to inhibit the growth of certain gut bacteria and promote the growth of others and are associated with beneficial health effects. The other important fact to note, though, is that polyphenols are also found in high levels in fruits, vegetables, coffee and tea, so red wine isn't a necessary dietary supplement to get more of them in your diet."

'Polyphenol' is one of those buzzwords that is often thrown around, but what does it mean? A polyphenol is a natural chemical found in some plant-based foods, from fruits and vegetables to coffee, chocolate and even red wine! Polyphenols are mini superheroes – they fight against damage caused by free radicals (a lot of this damage is an essential part of your body's processes). Polyphenols are like your microbes' cheerleaders – they help your microbes be their best selves by making them more efficient and feed those responsible for producing short-chain fatty acids.

Is a big session really worse than a couple of glasses at home?

"The other important factor to consider is the amount of alcohol consumed in one sitting. For red wine, only a couple of glasses a week was required to see the benefits in gut bacteria described opposite. In fact, there is good evidence that binge drinking – in this case a binge is more than 6 units for women or 8 units for men (a large glass of wine has 3 units, a shot has 1 unit) – leads to increased intestinal permeability (or 'leaky gut') and increased inflammatory proteins in the blood (head over to page 44 for more on this). This is probably due to a direct effect of one of the metabolites of alcohol, called acetaldehyde having a direct effect on the gut lining. Over time, it's possible that repeated inflammatory 'hits' may lead to chronic inflammation, which is linked to a number of chronic diseases, including mental health conditions. It's difficult to say how long it takes to recover fully from a binge, but our experiments with the BBC's *Horizon* ('Is Binge Drinking Really That Bad?' in 2015) suggest it takes at least a week, probably two. It's also important to say that regular, low-level drinking also leads to many other negative health consequences, such as an increased risk of cancer, but does not have the same effect on gut leakiness."

What is it that gives us the hangover?

"As mentioned above, acetaldehyde is one of the intermediate compounds generated in the metabolism of alcohol. Usually, acetaldehyde is broken down in the liver by an enzyme called aldehyde dehydrogenase. But this enzyme has a finite capacity and if it becomes saturated by excess alcohol during a binge, then acetaldehyde can start to accumulate. Acetaldehyde can cause nausea and flushing, contributing to some of the symptoms of a hangover (the other symptoms are probably because of leaky gut). So, one way to stop acetaldehyde accumulation is to slow down your drinking, helping to ensure that the enzymes metabolizing the alcohol can keep pace."

gut
cookin'

chapter 3

a note on dietary requirements

Before we get started, a little word on how you can change the recipes in this book to suit your dietary needs or allergy requirements.

Gluten: All the recipes in this book can be made gluten-free, using the following alternatives:

- Gluten-free flour, rice flour, gram flour

- Tamari (gluten-free) instead of soy sauce

- Gluten-free stock cubes

- Oats (while they don't contain gluten themselves, they are often processed in a factory that may have handled gluten – always check the label)

- Flavoured tofu and some plant-based alternative products

Gluten comes in many forms, from white flour to a spelt sourdough – if you don't need to remove it from your diet, think about variety; make sure you mix it up with different grains, like rye or spelt.

Dairy-free: Where we use dairy kefir or yogurt, you can swap for a dairy-free alternative (such as coconut kefir).

Swap cheese for nutritional yeast or vegan cheese (or you can omit altogether).

Swap dairy milks for plant-based milks – the choice is endless (coconut, oat, almond, soya and cashew). Look for ones that don't have lots of thickeners and stabilizers in.

Eggs: In baking, you can use a 'flax' egg – a tablespoon of flaxseed and a tablespoon of water. Add to recipes as you would an egg. Note – this doesn't make a poached egg substitute!

Food hygiene

How to prep, store and use in a safe way

It's all well and good knowing how to cook but we also want to help you with some practical tips to minimize food waste, reduce the risk of food poisoning (always a win), and encourage good habits when it comes to storing food.

AND before you get going... a bit of food hygiene (very important where microbes are involved).

Before you start: Before prepping and eating, ensure you wash your hands with soap and water (including any little people involved).

It may sound simple but many of us forget. Make sure you've got a clear surface wiped down with soapy water before you start. We always find it handy to get everything out of the cupboard/fridge/freezer before we start and have our equipment primed and ready (and wash this too before fermenting).

Wash: Wash all vegetables and fruit under cold water and, if they are particularly muddy, give them a good scrub.

Contamination: Minimize cross-contamination of raw and cooked meat and fish as these may contain potentially harmful microbes.

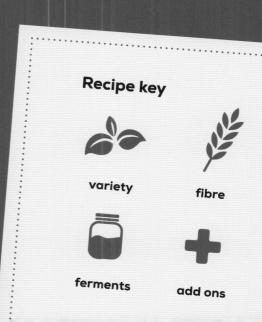

Recipe key

variety

fibre

ferments

add ons

spice up your life

Cupboards full of spices and don't know which spice girls to put in the band? Here's a handy guide to get them singing harmoniously together.

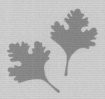

coriander

♥ curries
♥ salsa

+ ginger
+ garlic
+ chilli
+ fennel
+ cinnamon
+ turmeric

mint

♥ aubergine
♥ fruits

+ basil
+ cumin
+ ginger
+ oregano
+ parsley
+ thyme

sage

♥ stuffing
♥ tomatoes

+ garlic
+ paprika
+ parsley
+ thyme

basil

♥ tomatoes
♥ soups

+ paprika
+ garlic
+ oregano
+ rosemary
+ thyme

parsley

- ♥ fish
- ♥ salads

- ✚ basil
- ✚ garlic
- ✚ paprika
- ✚ mint

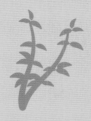

thyme

- ♥ chicken
- ♥ stews
- ♥ veg

- ✚ basil
- ✚ garlic
- ✚ nutmeg
- ✚ oregano
- ✚ rosemary

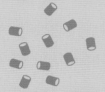

chives

- ♥ avocado
- ♥ salads
- ♥ cold plates

- ✚ fennel
- ✚ mint
- ✚ parsley
- ✚ sage
- ✚ thyme

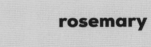

rosemary

- ♥ root veg
- ♥ stews

- ✚ garlic
- ✚ mint
- ✚ parsley
- ✚ sage
- ✚ thyme

oregano

- ♥ pasta
- ♥ tomatoes

- ✚ basil
- ✚ cumin
- ✚ garlic
- ✚ rosemary
- ✚ sage
- ✚ thyme

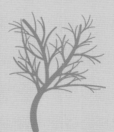

dill

- ♥ cabbage
- ♥ potatoes
- ♥ fish

- ✚ basil
- ✚ garlic
- ✚ cumin
- ✚ ginger
- ✚ turmeric

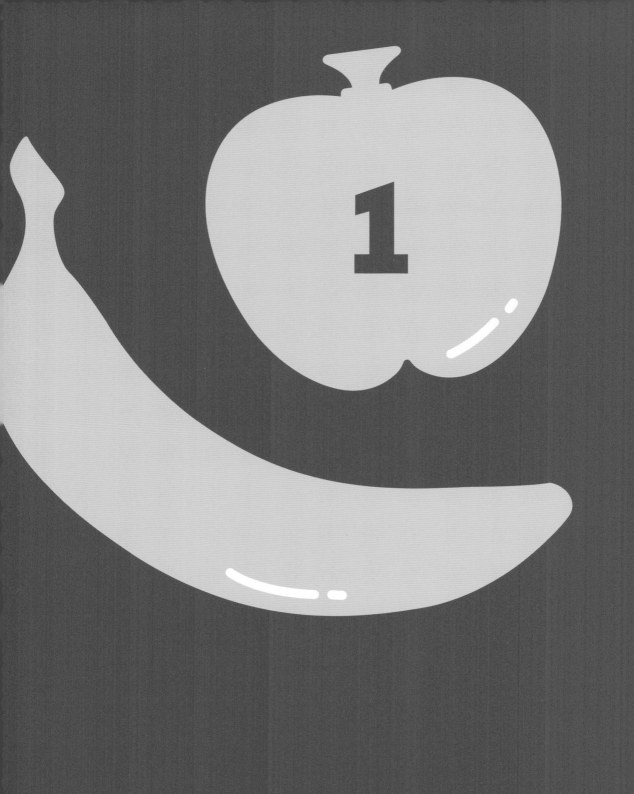

breakfast
and brunch

overnight oats

This brekkie is truly for EVERYONE, couldn't be easier to make and can add all your favourite toppings to suit your tastes! What's not to love – a great start to your day! Alana x

10 minutes | Serves 1

9.3g per portion

minimum 4

milk kefir

40g (1½ oz) oats

150ml (5 fl oz) milk kefir, (see also page 264), yogurt or milk *(dairy, plant, nut or other milk)*

1 apple, grated *(skin on)*

1–2 tsp nut butter *(such as peanut, almond or cashew)* or mixed seeds *(pumpkin, sunflower, seame, flaxseed or linseed)*

1 tsp ground cinnamon

allergens: *gluten, milk, nuts (make gluten- and dairy-free using alternatives and omit the nuts if needed)*

1. Place all the ingredients into a 500ml (18-fl oz) jar, stir well, cover with a screw-top lid and place in the fridge for a minimum of 2 hours or ideally overnight.

2. When the oats have hydrated and thickened the mixture, pour the contents of the jar into your bowl. Add the toppings of your choice just before serving.

Store in the fridge for up to 4 days.

FLAVOUR COMBOS

Fibre – 8.5g
carrot cake – Swap the grated apple for a grated carrot (skin on) and add 1 teaspoon honey or maple syrup and swap the ground cinnamon for 1 teaspoon allspice. Swap the nut butter or mixed seeds for a handful of chopped walnuts to top.

Fibre – 9g
blueberry cobbler – Swap the grated apple for a handful of blueberries and add 1 tablespoon chia seeds.

Fibre – 9g
spiced pear – Swap the grated apple with a chopped pear (skin on). Swap the ground cinnamon for 1 teaspoon allspice and swap the nut butter or mixed seeds for a handful of chopped walnuts to top.

Fibre – 7.5g

strawberries and cream – Swap the grated apple with a handful of chopped strawberries and top with a spoonful of milk kefir yogurt.

Fibre – 12g

cherry chocolate – Swap the grated apple with 80g (3 oz) cherry chia jam (see below). Swap the cinnamon for 1 tablespoon cacao powder.

Fibre – 10.3g

peanut butter and strawberry chia jam – Top with 2 tablespoons strawberry chia jam (see below) and 1 tablespoon peanut butter (see below).

....

FRUIT CHIA JAM

15 minutes | Servings 4

strawberries
(4.8g per 80g)
cherries
(2.9g per 80g)
mixed berries
(3.9g per 80g)
raspberries
(7g per 80g)

300g (10½ oz) fresh or frozen fruit, such as strawberries, cherries, mixed berries or raspberries

2 tbsp chia seeds

1. Place the fruit in a small saucepan over a low heat, stirring occasionally, until it begins to break down. Use a spoon to mash the fruit to your desired consistency, adding a splash of water to loosen if required. Stir in the chia seeds until combined. Remove from the heat and leave to cool for 5 minutes.

Once cool, store fruit chia jam in the fridge in an airtight container for up to 4 days.

....

NUT BUTTER

25 minutes | Servings 10–12

peanuts
(1.5g per tbsp)
almonds
(3.3g per tbsp)
cashews
(1g per tbsp)

250g (9 oz) nuts, such as peanuts, almonds or cashews

pinch of sea salt

1. Preheat the oven to 180°C fan/200°C/400°F/ gas mark 6. Scatter the nuts over a large baking tray and toast in the oven for 10–15 minutes until golden. Remove from the oven and leave to cool. Transfer the nuts to a blender with the salt. Blend for 5–10 minutes until you're left with a smooth nut butter.

Store nut butter at room temperature in an airtight container for up to 2 weeks.

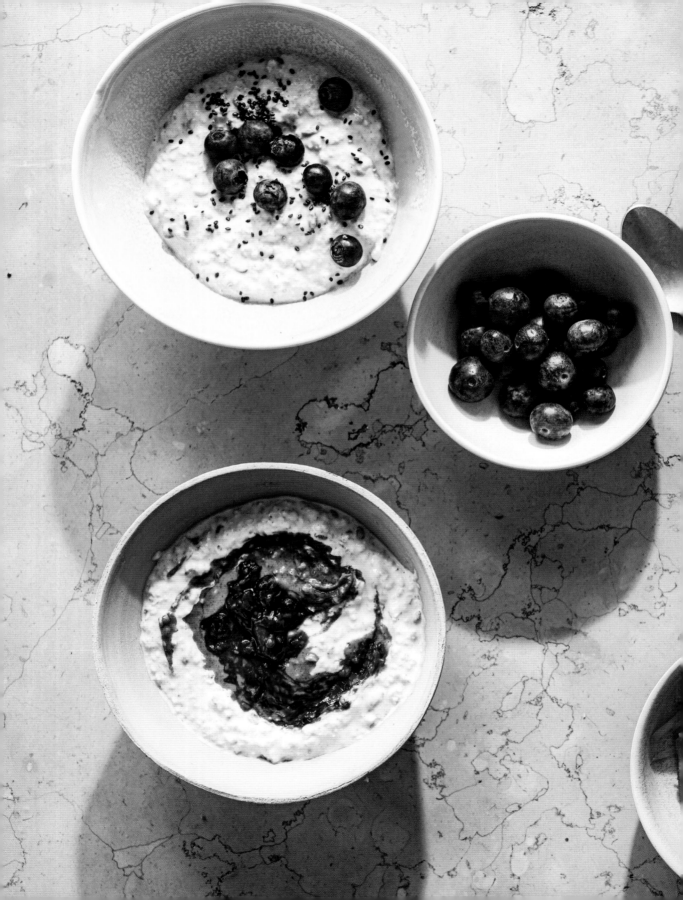

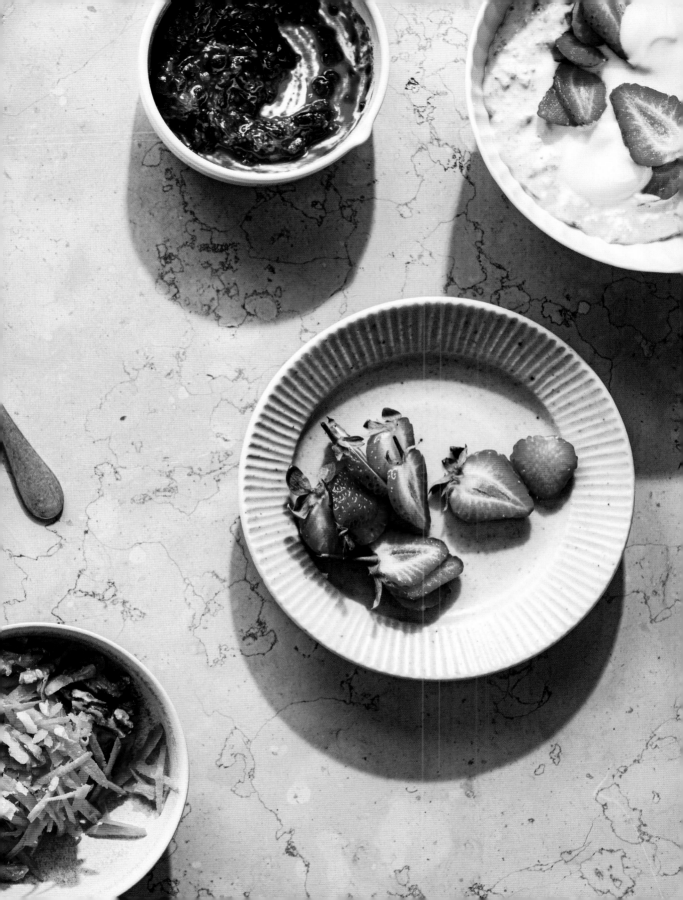

spiced green pancakes

Who said pancakes gotta be sweet? I love these for a weekend brunch or a lazy late lunch. Excellent with a spicy Bloody Mary ;) Lisa x

50 minutes | Serves 4
(including 20 minutes resting time)

 7.7g per portion

 11

 milk kefir

allergens: *gluten, cow's milk (if using), eggs*

PANCAKES

1 garlic clove, peeled

handful of fresh coriander

handful of spinach

½ tsp ground cumin

½ tsp ground cardamom

100ml (3½ fl oz) milk or oat milk, plus extra if needed

125g (4½ oz) spelt flour

2 large eggs

1–2 tbsp butter

salt and pepper

TOPPING

1 avocado, cut into chunks

2 spring onions, finely sliced

2 handfuls of spinach

2 tbsp milk kefir (home-made, see page 264, or shop-bought)

1 x 200g (7 oz) can of sweetcorn, drained

½ tbsp chilli flakes

squeeze of lemon juice

1. Put the garlic, coriander, spinach, cumin and cardamom in a blender and blitz to a smooth green paste. Add a splash of the milk or oat milk to loosen if needed.

2. Add the flour to a large mixing bowl and create a well, then add the eggs, slowly whisking them into the flour. Add a pinch of salt and stir, then gradually add the milk, followed by the green paste and whisk to combine. Leave to rest for 20 minutes at room temperature.

3. Put all the topping ingredients in a mixing bowl, season with salt and pepper and stir to combine.

4. Melt the butter in a 20cm (8 in) non-stick frying pan over a medium heat. Once hot, whisk the batter, then ladle 60ml (4 tbsp) into the pan. Cook for 2 minutes, then flip and cook for a further minute. Transfer to a plate and repeat, serve with the mixed topping.

Store any leftover pancakes in an airtight container in the fridge for 3–4 days. The topping is best prepared and served immediately.

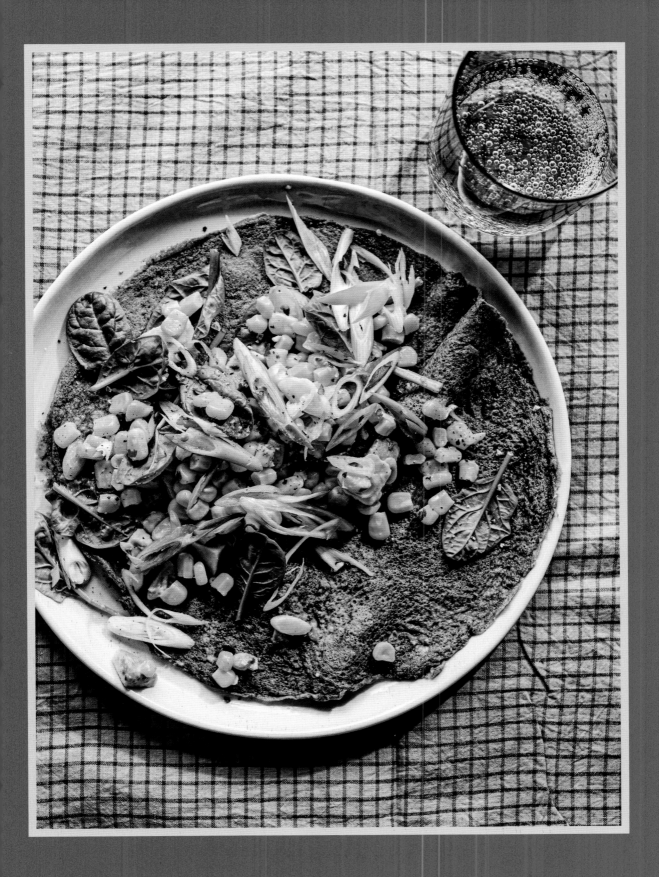

sourdough french toast with mixed berry compote

This is a tooty fruity but not-too-sweet twist on traditional French toast (or eggy bread!) using sourdough. Frozen berries are a quick way to add variety and great for the winter months when berries tend to be out of season. Lisa x

20 minutes | Serves 2

6g per portion

minimum 4

sourdough and milk kefir yogurt

allergens: *gluten, cow's milk (if using), egg*

1 egg

50ml (2 fl oz) milk *(dairy, plant, nut or other milk)*

1 tsp ground cinnamon or allspice

zest and juice of ½ lemon

2 slices of sourdough *(homemade, see page 252, or shop-bought)*

200g (7 oz) frozen mixed berries

20ml (4 tsp) water

1 tbsp butter

2 tbsp mixed seeds *(pumpkin, sunflower, sesame, flaxseed or linseed)*

2 tbsp honey or maple syrup *(optional)*

1 tsp coconut flakes *(optional)*

milk kefir yogurt *(homemade, see page 264, or shop-bought), to serve (optional)*

Fibre and Variety – add a side of chocolate hummus *(see pages 216–217)*
Ferments – add a spoonful of milk kefir yogurt *(see page 264)*

1. Whisk the egg, milk and cinnamon or allspice together in a shallow bowl. Stir in the lemon zest. Add the sourdough slices to the mixture and leave to soak for 2 minutes, then turn over and soak for a further 2 minutes.

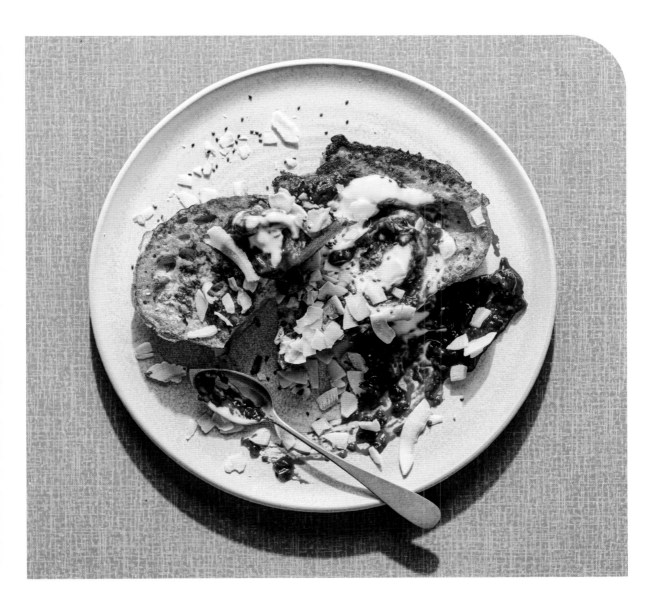

2. Place a small saucepan over a low heat, add the mixed berries and the lemon juice and water. Cook for 5 minutes until the berries have softened.

3. Heat the butter in a non-stick frying pan over a medium heat. Add the soaked sourdough, cook for 2 minutes until golden brown and then flip to cook the other side for a further 2 minutes.

4. Serve the sourdough toast topped with the mixed berry compote, mixed seeds, honey or maple syrup, coconut flakes and a dollop of milk kefir yogurt (if using).

Store any leftover compote in an airtight container in the fridge for up to 4 days.

bubble and squeak

A classic, PLUS if you leave your mash to cool completely, the potato starch becomes magic resistant starch with prebiotic properties for your good ole gut bugs. Lisa x

40 minutes | Serves 2
(including 20 minutes
resting time)

 minimum 7g per portion without toppings

 minimum 4

 see topping suggestions

allergens: *cow's milk, if using milk kefir yogurt; fish, if using smoked salmon*

2 large handfuls of mixed vegetables, such as Brussels sprouts, cabbage *(any colour)*, kale or cavolo nero

1 parsnip *(skin on)*, roughly grated

4 spring onions, sliced

500g (14 oz) leftover mashed potato or grated potato *(skin on)*

1 tbsp olive oil

salt and pepper

TOPPINGS

MILK KEFIR YOGURT, SMOKED SALMON AND FRESH CHIVES

4 tbsp milk kefir yogurt *(homemade, see page 264, or shop-bought)*

120g (4¼ oz) smoked salmon

handful of fresh chives, roughly chopped

HUMMUS, SAUERKRAUT AND FRESH PARSLEY

50g (1¾ oz) hummus *(home-made, see page 216, or shop-bought)*

50g (1¾ oz) sauerkraut *(homemade, see page 256, or shop-bought)*

handful of fresh flat-leaf parsley, roughly chopped

AVOCADO, KIMCHI AND FRESH CORIANDER

1 ripe avocado, sliced

50g (1¾ oz) kimchi *(home-made, see page 260, or shop-bought)*

handful of fresh coriander, roughly chopped

Mashed potato

1. Roughly chop the potato (skin on) into cubes. Bring a medium saucepan of salted water to the boil. Add the potatoes and cook for 20–25 minutes until tender. Remove from the heat, drain and steam-dry for 5 minutes. Roughly mash using a potato masher, then rest for 20 minutes to cool completely for magic resistant starch.

2. Wash and finely shred the mixed vegetables. If using kale or cavolo nero, remove the woody stalks first. If using grated potato, squeeze out any excess liquid from the potatoes.

3. Add 1 tsp of the olive oil to a medium non-stick frying pan over a medium heat. Add the shredded veg and cook for 2–4 minutes until it begins to wilt. Remove from the heat and set aside. In a mixing bowl, combine the mashed potato, grated parsnip, spring onions and vegetables. Season well.

4. Add the remaining olive oil to the medium non-stick frying pan and return to a medium heat. Add the potato mixture and press down, using a wooden spoon or spatula, so it covers the base of the pan. Cook for 4 minutes, then fold the crispy bottom back into the mixture. Press the mixture back down and cook for a further 5–7 minutes until golden brown, then flip and cook the other side until golden brown. If the mixture breaks when flipping, press it down again. Top with one of our topping suggestions.

Store any leftovers in the fridge for up to 2 days.

creamy mushrooms on sourdough

I used to think the cashew soaking was a FAFF but it's well worth it to pimp up that toast. Lisa x

20 minutes | Serves 4

+ 15 minutes to pre-soak cashews

 8g per portion

 minimum 6

 sourdough

allergens: *nuts (cashews), gluten, cow's milk*

50g (1¾ oz) cashews

200g (7 oz) shredded kale

1 tbsp olive oil

1 x 400g (14 oz) can of cannellini or butter beans, drained and rinsed

50ml (2 fl oz) water

1 tbsp salted butter

1 shallot, finely diced

1 garlic clove, crushed

handful of fresh flat-leaf parsley, stalks finely chopped and leaves kept whole

400g (14 oz) mushrooms, such as button, chestnut, portobello finely sliced

4 slices of sourdough

salt and pepper

1. Place the cashews in a bowl and soak in boiling water for 15 minutes, then drain.

2. Preheat the oven to 180°C fan/200°C/400°F/ gas mark 6. Spread the kale over a baking tray and drizzle with the oil, scrunching to ensure it's evenly coated. Season and cook for 10–15 minutes.

3. Place the soaked cashews, beans and water in a food processor and purée until smooth. Thin out with more water if required. Season with salt and pepper.

4. In a medium frying pan, heat the butter and cook the shallot for 3–5 minutes until softened. Add the garlic and parsley stalks and cook together for 1 minute. Add the mushrooms and cook for a further 3–5 minutes. Add the cashew and bean sauce and heat through.

5. Serve the mushrooms on toasted sourdough, topped with the crispy kale and parsley leaves.

Best eaten straight away.

veggie brunch

I love doing this if I'm feeling a bit swanky on a Saturday – and such a great way to use up my greens. We stuck with veggie here, but I also like to add a couple of sausages. Lisa x

20 minutes | Serves 2
with the TGS baked beans (make in advance)

8.4g with TGS baked beans per portion

minimum 9

sourdough

allergens: *cow's milk, gluten (if using sourdough), eggs (if using)*

1 tsp butter
150g (7 oz) mushrooms (*any variety*), roughly chopped
400g (7 oz) baked beans (*homemade, see page 150 or shop-bought*)
2 handfuls of greens (*such as spinach, cavolo nero or kale*), shredded
120g (5¾ oz) halloumi, cut into 1cm (½ in) slices
salt and pepper

TO SERVE (OPTIONAL)
2 eggs (*the fresher the better*)
1 tbsp white wine vinegar
2 slices of toasted sourdough (*homemade, see page 252, or shop-bought*)

Fibre – a handful of mixed seeds
Variety – use a mixed variety of mushrooms
Ferments – add a side of sourdough toast or olives

1. Add the butter to a large non-stick pan over a medium-high heat, add the mushrooms and brown for 3–5 minutes.

2. Meanwhile, add the baked beans to a small saucepan and heat through over a medium-low heat. Add the greens to the mushrooms, reduce the heat and cook for a further 3 minutes, stirring occasionally. Add a splash of water, if required. Season, then push the mixture to the edge of the pan and add the halloumi. Cook for 2 minutes on each side until golden brown.

3. If you're having eggs; while the halloumi is frying, fill a small saucepan with water and bring to a rolling boil. Add the vinegar and crack the eggs carefully into the water. Cook for 2–3 minutes, then remove with a slotted spoon. Serve with the veggie brunch on toasted sourdough.

Store any leftovers in an airtight container in the fridge for up to 3 days.

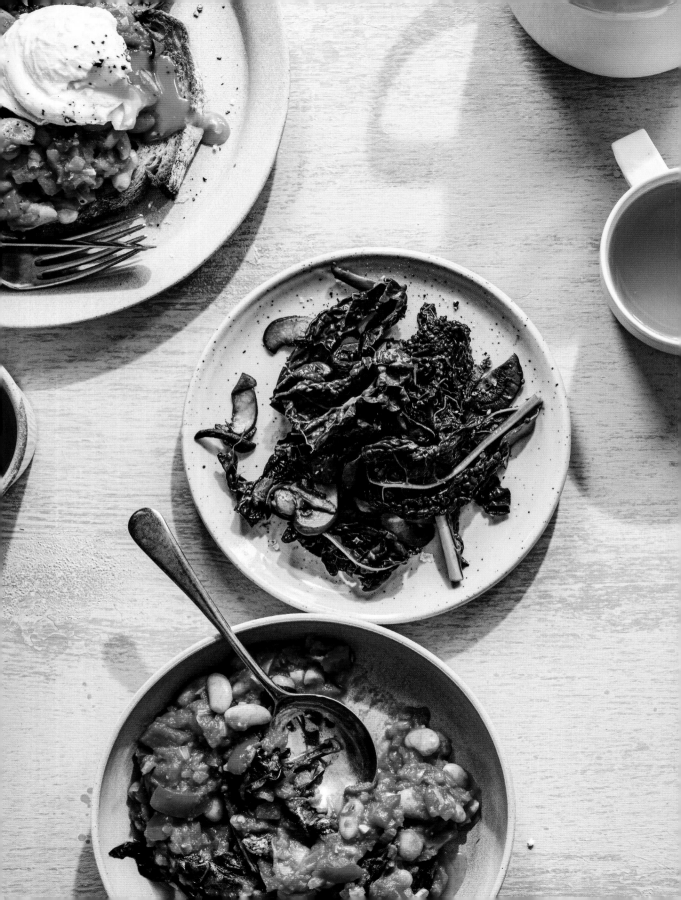

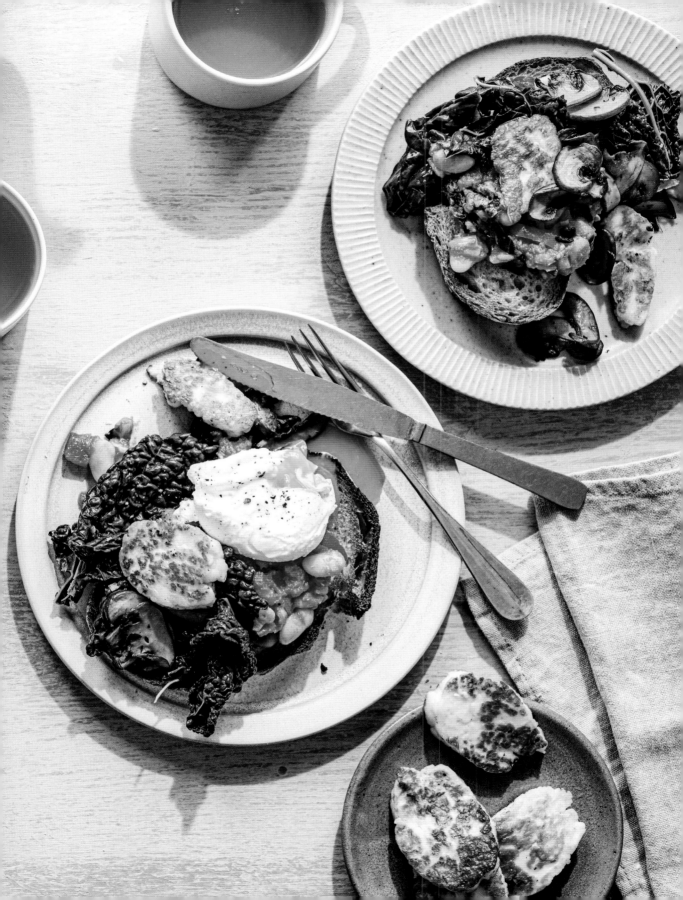

'gut' baked beans

Our mum used to always sing the 'beans beans, good for your heart, the more you eat...' etc. etc. whilst serving us baked beans and now we've got our own rootin' tootin' version. Alana x

40 minutes | Serves 4

5.4g per portion

minimum 7

sourdough

1 tbsp olive oil

1 onion (*white or red*), roughly chopped

2 peppers (*red or yellow*), deseeded and roughly chopped

2 garlic cloves, roughly chopped

1 heaped tsp paprika or smoked paprika (*for a smoky twist*)

pinch of chilli flakes (*optional*)

1 x 400g (14 oz) can of tomatoes (*any type*)

1 x 400g (14 oz) can of white beans, such as butter beans or haricot, drained and rinsed

salt and pepper

toasted sourdough (*homemade, see page 252, or shop-bought*)

a baked potato or veggie brunch (*see page 147*), to serve

Fibre – add 2 handfuls of frozen spinach for the final 5 minutes of cooking

Variety – use a mixed variety can of beans

1. Heat the olive oil in a saucepan over a medium-high heat. Add the onion and a pinch of salt and cook for 5 minutes until softened, stirring occasionally.

2. Add the peppers and cook for 2 minutes. Add the garlic, paprika and chilli flakes (if using) and cook for 2 minutes.

3. Add the tomatoes, then swill a splash of water around the can and add this to the pan too. Bring to the boil, then reduce the heat and simmer for 15 minutes.

4. Remove from the heat and use a stick blender to create a smooth sauce. Season to taste. Return to the heat, stir in the beans and cook until warmed through.

5. Serve on top of toasted sourdough, a baked potato or with our veggie brunch.

Store in an airtight container in the fridge for up to 3 days.

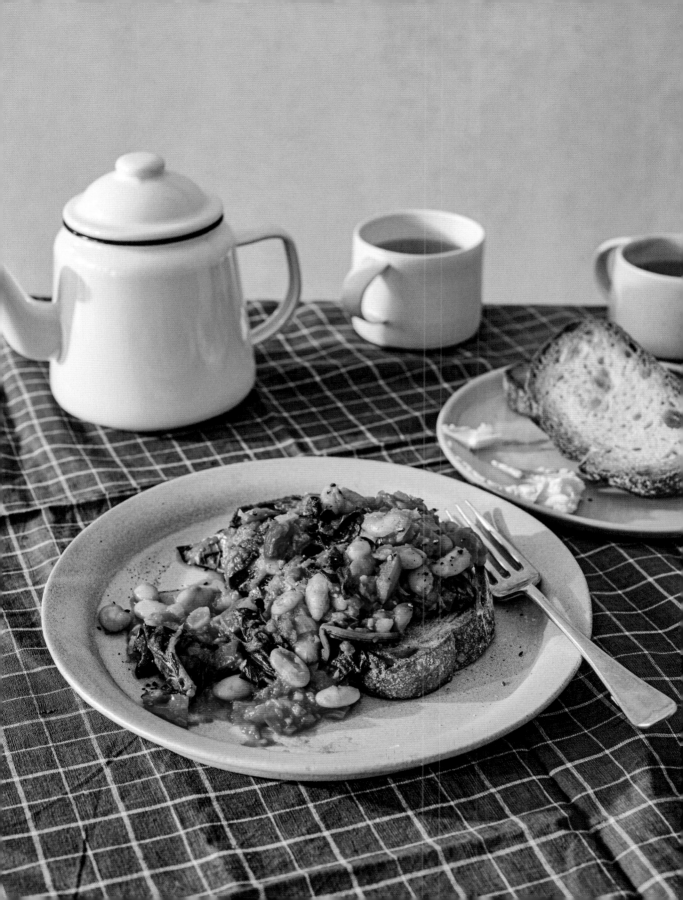

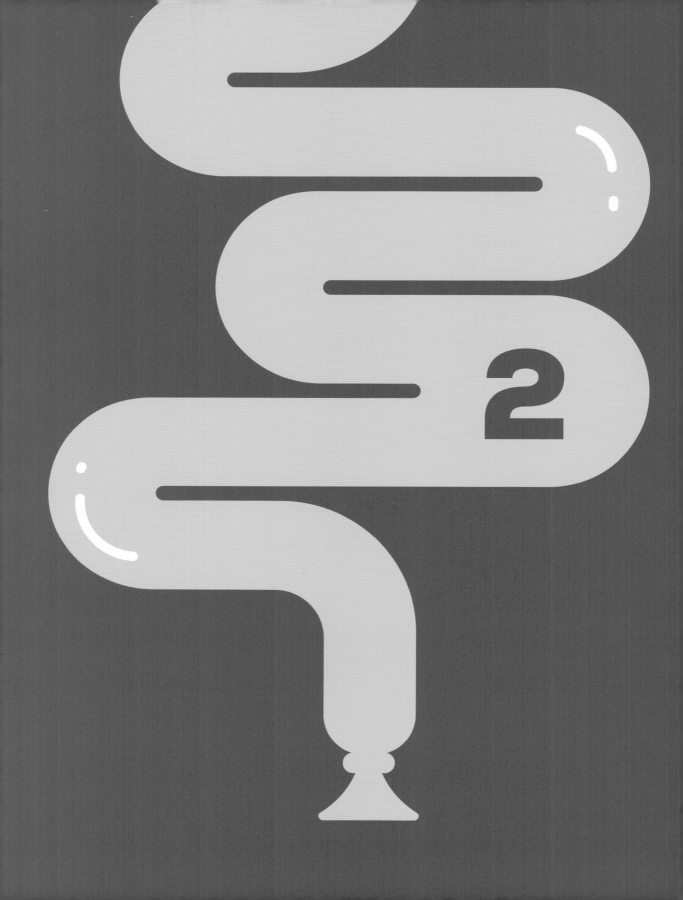

a gut lunch

chicken goujon caesar salad with fibre cracker croutons

Love this if I've got pals round and want to make a wee alfresco dining effort without just shoving packets of goujons in the oven... My cheeky twist is to use almonds to make a crunchy coating. I usually make a full batch of fibre crackers to keep, but they're usually all munched as I'm cooking ha! Lisa x

1 hour 10 minutes | Serves 2
(including fibre crackers)

8.6g with fibre cracker per portion

minimum 9 *(based on 3 different types in the mixed leaf bag)*

milk kefir yogurt

½ fibre crackers mixture
(*see page 157*)
2 skinless chicken breasts
30g (1¾ oz) ground almonds
1 tsp paprika
1 egg
2 romaine lettuces
2 handfuls of mixed leaves
salt and pepper

DRESSING
20g (1¾ oz) Parmesan cheese
1 small garlic clove, grated
2 canned anchovy fillets, finely chopped
squeeze of lemon juice
4 tbsp milk kefir yogurt
(*homemade, see page 264, or shop-bought*)
1 tbsp extra virgin olive oil

allergens: *nuts (almonds), egg, fish, cow's milk*

Fibre – top with 100g (3½ oz) jarred artichoke, roughly chopped
Variety – a handful of sliced cherry tomatoes
Ferments – top with a handful of olives

1. Preheat the oven to 180°C fan/200°C/400°F/gas mark 6 and line two baking trays with baking paper.

2. Begin by mixing all the ingredients for the fibre crackers together.

Recipe continued overleaf

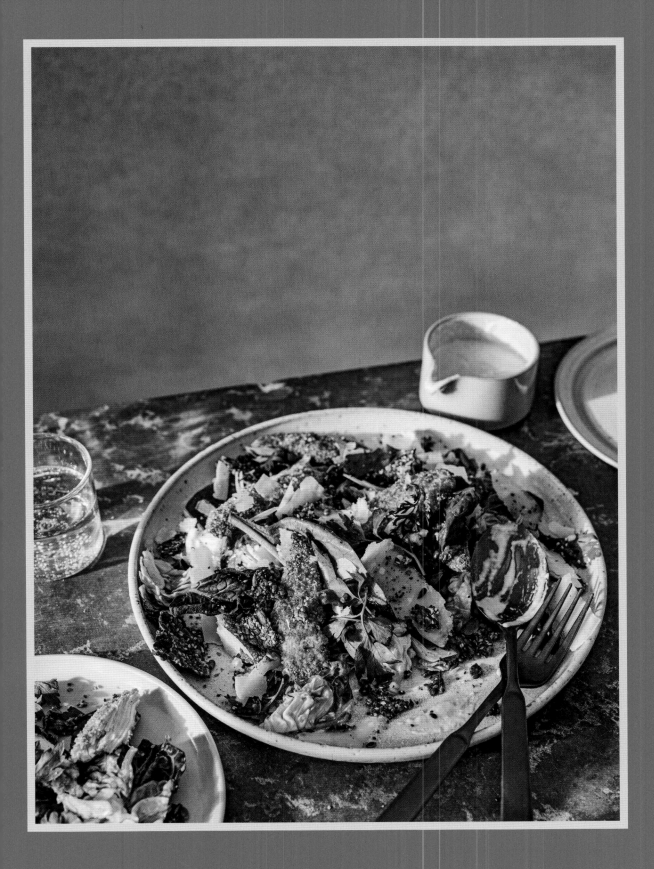

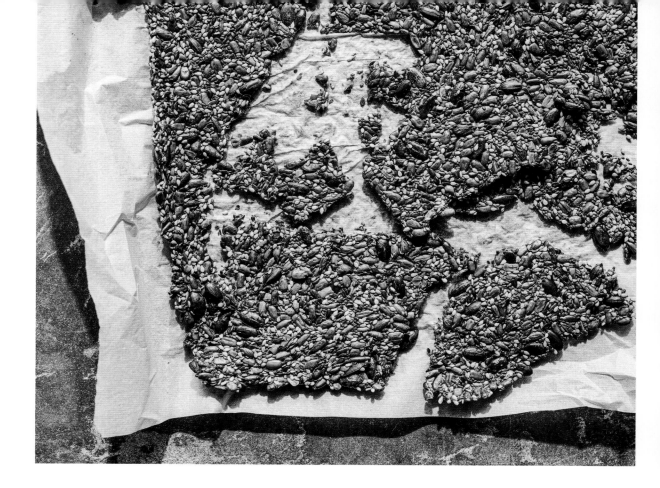

3. While the fibre cracker mixture is soaking, prepare the chicken goujons. Using a sharp knife, cut the chicken into strips. Mix the ground almonds and paprika in a shallow bowl and season well. In another shallow bowl, whisk the egg. Coat the chicken goujons one by one in the beaten egg and then the almond-paprika mixture. Arrange on one of the lined baking trays.

4. Once the fibre cracker mixture has thickened, spread it thinly over the second lined baking tray until it's around 5mm (¼-in) thick. Bake for 25 minutes, then add the tray of chicken to the oven too and bake both for a further 25 minutes, turning the chicken halfway through cooking.

5. To make the dressing, finely grate half the Parmesan and add to the milk kefir yogurt in a jug with the anchovies, garlic, lemon juice and olive oil. Stir well to combine and season to taste.

6. Shred the lettuce and add to a large mixing bowl with the mixed leaves and coat in the dressing.

7. Crumble the fibre cracker and use a peeler to cut the remaining Parmesan into shavings.

8. To serve, top the leaves with the chicken goujons, sprinkle over the crumbled fibre cracker and Parmesan shavings.

Best served immediately.

fibre crackers

I buy huge bags of nuts and seeds and prep loads on a Sunday to make crackers for dipping and crumbling onto soups and salads... moreish beyond belief... Lisa x

**20 mins prep +
50 minutes cooking** | **Makes 10 crackers
5 portions**

65g (2¼ oz) sunflower seeds

50g (1¾ oz) pumpkin seeds

35g (1¼ oz) chia seeds

35g (1¼ oz) sesame seeds

20g (¾ oz) whole flaxseeds

½ tsp salt

180ml (6 fl oz) water

5.8g per portion

5

allergens: *sesame*

1. Preheat the oven to 180°C fan/200°C/400°F/ gas mark 6 and line a medium baking tray with baking paper.

2. Mix all the ingredients together and leave for 15 minutes for the chia seeds to soak up the water. Once the mixture has thickened, spread thinly over the lined baking tray until around 5mm (¼-in) thick. Bake for 50 minutes. If the cracker doesn't feel crisp after 50 minutes, return to the oven for a further 5–10 minutes.

3. Remove from the oven and leave to cool before breaking into crackers.

Store in an airtight container for up to a week.

Fibre – top with hummus *(see page 216)*
Variety – top with a handful of rocket
Ferments – top with sauerkraut or kimchi *(see pages 256 and 260).*

oMEGA salad

Tuna salad is my go-to if grabbing lunch on the move, so this is a nourishing homemade version (much better in my opinion!). Genuinely so filling too... bring on the Omega 3! Alana x

30 minutes | Serves 4

10g per portion

minimum 9

olives

allergens: *fish, eggs*

4 eggs

200g (7 oz) baby new potatoes, halved

2 handfuls of green beans, trimmed

2 Little Gem lettuces

200g (7 oz) cherry or plum tomatoes

50g (1¾ oz) stoned olives

1 small red onion

handful of fresh flat-leaf parsley

1 x 400g (14 oz) can of chickpeas, drained and rinsed

2 handfuls of mixed leaves

2–3 tbsp extra virgin olive oil

100g (3½ oz) marinated white or canned anchovy fillets

squeeze of lemon juice

salt and pepper

1. To soft-boil the eggs, ensure the eggs are room temperature. Bring a medium saucepan of water to a rolling boil, add the eggs and set a timer for 6–7 minutes. Transfer the eggs to cold water to cool before peeling and cutting into quarters.

2. Heat a large saucepan of salted water over a high heat. Once the water is boiling, add the potatoes, reduce the heat and simmer for 15–20 minutes until tender. Add the green beans for the final 2 minutes. Drain and leave to steam-dry while you prepare the rest of the salad.

3. Remove the end of each lettuce and cut into quarters lengthways, halve the tomatoes and the olives, thinly slice the onion and roughly chop the parsley. Add to a large mixing bowl (except the olives) along with the chickpeas, cooked potatoes and green beans. Drizzle over the extra virgin olive oil, combine and season to taste.

+

Fibre – top with 2 tsp mixed seeds

Variety – add 2 handfuls of spinach leaves

Ferments – toss the salad in milk kefir yogurt (see page 264)

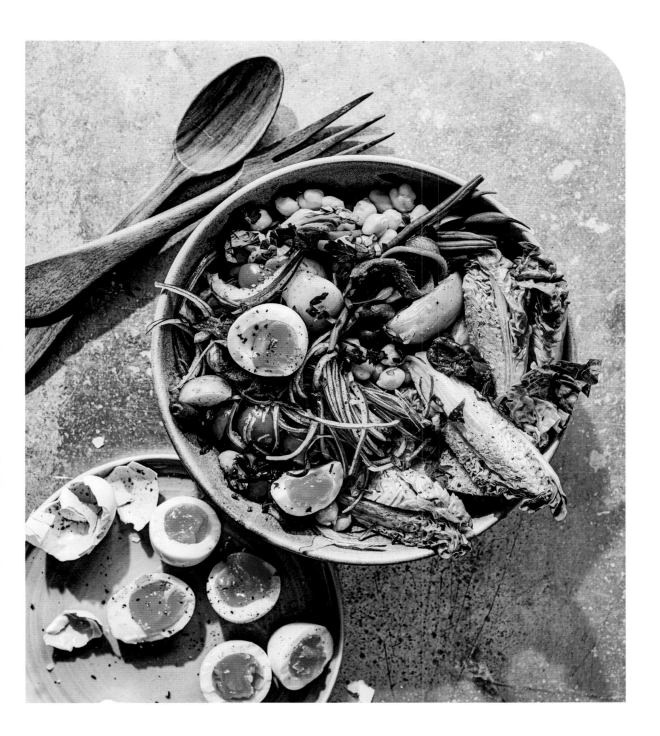

4. To serve, top the dressed salad with the quartered eggs, olives and anchovies. Finish with a squeeze of lemon juice.

Store any leftovers in an airtight container in the fridge for up to a day.

shredded brussels sprouts salad

I am FOREVER thinking up what to do with sprouts – my go-to was always pan-fried with pancetta and walnuts, but here's a cheeky non-Christmas alternative. Got a newfound love for them. Lisa x

20 minutes | Serves 4

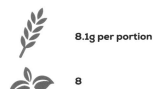

8.1g per portion

8

allergens: *milk (if using feta), nuts (walnuts)*

60g (2¼ oz) walnuts
100g (3½ oz) kale
1 fennel bulb
200g (7 oz) Brussels sprouts
handful of fresh flat-leaf parsley
2–3 tbsp extra virgin olive oil

400g (7 oz) cooked quinoa
zest and juice of ½ lemon
120g (2¾ oz) crumbled feta cheese *(optional)*
seeds of 1 pomegranate
salt and pepper

Fibre – top with crumbled fibre crackers *(see page 157)*
Variety – a side of hummus *(see page 216)*
Ferments – top with sauerkraut *(see page 256)*

1. Preheat the oven to 180°C fan/200°C/400°F/gas mark 6.

2. Scatter the walnuts over a baking tray and cook for 10 minutes until lightly toasted. Remove the woody stalks from the kale and roughly shred. Finely shred the fennel and Brussels sprouts. Roughly chop the parsley.

3. Add the kale to a mixing bowl along with 1 tablespoon of the olive oil and half the lemon juice. Season well and massage the kale leaves for 2–5 minutes until softened. Add the Brussels sprouts, fennel, quinoa and parsley. Gradually add the remaining lemon juice (checking the flavour as you add!) and the zest, remaining olive oil and season to taste.

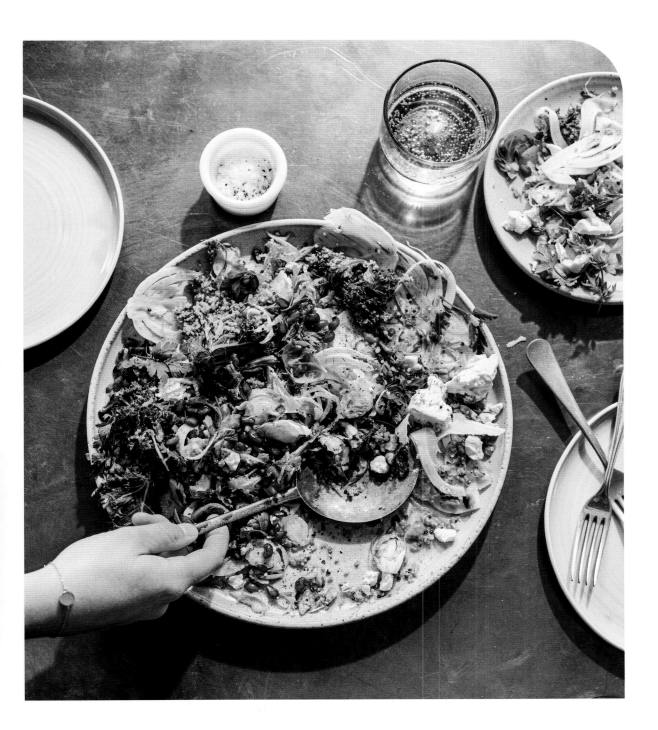

4. Roughly chop the toasted walnuts. Top the mixed salad with the crumbled feta (if using), chopped walnuts and pomegranate seeds.

Store any leftovers in an airtight container in the fridge for up to 3 days. Leftover walnuts will keep better stored at room temperature in an airtight container.

sunshine bowl

Colourful, quick summer in a bowl. Pre-cooked packet grains are great for this. Enough said. Lisa x

10 minutes | Serves 2

minimum 11g per portion

minimum 9

milk kefir yogurt

250g (5½ oz) pre-cooked grains *(freekeh, buckwheat, bulgur or brown rice)**

1 carrot *(skin on)*

1 pepper *(any colour)*, deseeded and sliced

handful of cherry tomatoes, halved

2 handfuls of baby spinach

4 tbsp milk kefir yogurt *(homemade, see page 264, or shop-bought)*

4 tbsp crunchy nut and seed mix *(see page 229)*

salt and pepper

allergens: *nuts (dependant on nut used in crunchy nut and seed topping), cow's milk*

1. Use a vegetable peeler to slice the carrot into ribbons lengthways.

2. Place the carrot, pepper and tomatoes in a mixing bowl along with the spinach and grains, stir in the milk kefir yogurt and season.

3. To serve, divide the grains and vegetable mixture between two shallow bowls and sprinkle with the crunchy nut and seed mix.

Store any leftover salad in the fridge for up to a day. The crunchy nut and seed topping is best stored at room temperature in an airtight container for up to 2 weeks.

Fibre – 1 sliced avocado
Variety – a side of green or black bean and lime hummus *(see pages 216–217)*
Ferments – top with kimchi or sauerkraut *(see pages 256 and 260)*

**Heat the mixed grains according to the packet instructions.*

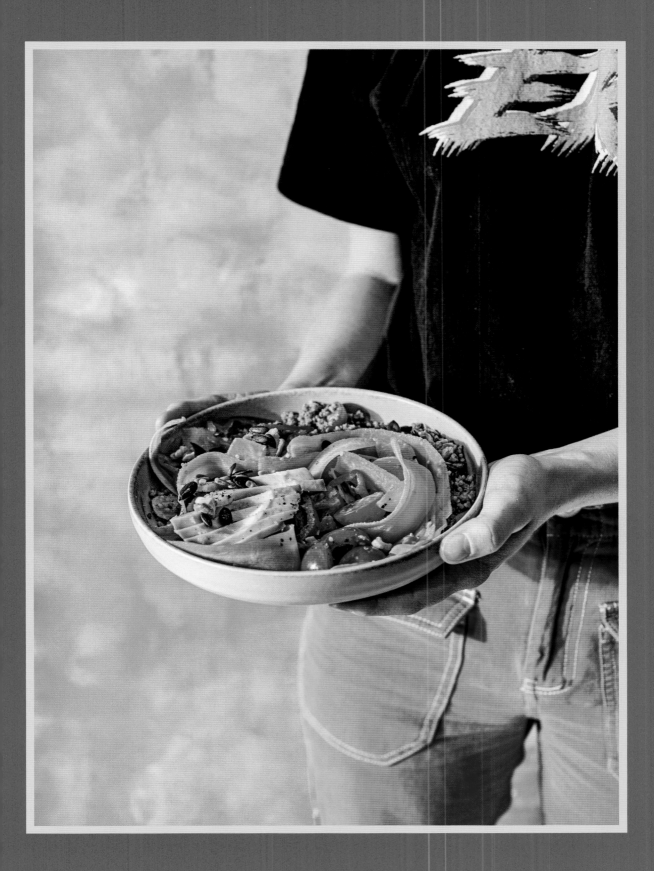

build your own plant-based traybake

Like Tetris, for veg. You do you. Lisa and Alana x

30 minutes | Serves 2

 Fibre – hummus *(see page 216)*
Variety – mixed whole grains or quinoa
Ferments – sauerkraut, kimchi or fermented hot sauce *(see pages 256, 260 and 227)*

BASE

choose 1 bean, pulse or veg

BEAN AND PULSES

1 packet or 400g (14-oz) can of cooked lentils

1 x 400g (14-oz) can of chickpeas

1 x 400g (14-oz) can of beans *(butter, haricot, black, cannellini, black-eyed, aduki)*

BASE VEG

butternut squash *(skin on)*, roughly chopped

sweet potato *(skin on)*, roughly chopped

parsnip *(skin on)*, roughly chopped

turnip, roughly chopped

swede, roughly chopped

carrot *(skin on)*, roughly chopped

PLANTS

choose at least 2

handful of tomatoes, halved

1 onion, roughly chopped *(any colour)*

1 pepper, roughly chopped *(any colour)*

handful of broccoli, roughly chopped

handful of radishes, halved

handful of asparagus, woody ends removed

handful of green beans, trimmed

1 aubergine, roughly chopped

handful of baby corn

handful of mushrooms *(any variety)*, halved

1 courgette, roughly chopped

handful of grapes

handful of frozen broccoli, peas or cauliflower

FLAVOUR

choose at least 1 (*see spice pairings infographic, pages 132–133*)

1–2 tsp dried spices (*ground cumin or coriander, sumac, paprika, smoked paprika*)

1 tbsp dried herbs (*oregano, thyme, rosemary, sage*)

citrus zest and juice (*lemon, lime or orange*)

garlic cloves, crushed or smashed

dried or fresh chilli

....

TOPPINGS

choose at least 1

2 tbsp crunchy seed and nut mix (*see page 229*)

2 tbsp mixed seeds (*pumpkin, sunflower, sesame, flaxseed or linseed*)

handful of stoned olives

2 tbsp mixed nuts (*walnuts, cashews, almonds, hazelnuts or pistachios*)

handful of mixed fresh herbs (*flat-leaf parsley, basil, coriander or chives*)

sliced avocado

60g (2¼ oz) crumbled feta

handful of leaves (*rocket, spinach, watercress or a mixture*)

extra virgin olive oil

2–3 tbsp olive oil, to cook

....

1. Preheat the oven to 200°C fan/220°C/425°F/gas mark 7. If using base veg, bring a pan of salted water to the boil, then parboil for 5–7 minutes, drain and steam-dry for 2 minutes.

2. Add the base beans, pulses or veg, your selection of plants and 2–3 tablespoons olive oil to a medium baking tray. Stir to coat the ingredients in the oil. Add the flavouring, if using spices or herbs or zest, scatter evenly and stir to combine. Finish with a squeeze of citrus, if using. Cook for 15 minutes, then give everything a good stir. Return to the oven and cook for a further 10–15 minutes until everything is slightly golden and tender.

3. Once cooked, serve the traybake with your selection of toppings.

Store any leftovers in the fridge for up to 3 days.

one-pot chicken noodles

Every time I think about ordering a takeaway, I make this instead – so yum!
Just make sure you don't spill all the peppercorns on the floor (like I did…) Alana x

1 hour | Serves 4

 minimum 7g per portion

 minimum 6

 miso paste

allergens: *sesame (if using sesame oil), soya, gluten (see miso paste), egg (check noodle packaging)*

 Fibre – use wholegrain noodles such as soba
Variety – top with crunchy nut and seed mix *(see page 229)*
Ferments – top with kimchi *(see page 260)*

250g (9 oz) dried soba noodles

1 tbsp sesame oil or light olive oil

4 shallots, roughly chopped

4 garlic cloves, smashed

7.5cm (3-in) piece of fresh ginger, unpeeled and roughly sliced

1 small chicken, weighing 1–1.2kg (2 lb 4 oz–2 lb 11 oz)

1.2 litres (2 pints) water

2 carrots *(skin on)*, roughly chopped

10 whole peppercorns

2–3 tbsp miso paste *(double check for wheat, barley or rye if need to avoid gluten)*

120g baby or frozen spinach

salt

TOPPING

1 tbsp sesame oil or light olive oil

400g (14 oz) mixed vegetables, such as broccoli, green beans, frozen peas or sweetcorn, spring greens, kale, pak choi, asparagus, roughly chopped as necessary

1 red chilli, deseeded and finely sliced

1 garlic clove, finely sliced

handful of fresh coriander, roughly chopped

squeeze of lime juice

1. To make the stock, add 1 tablespoon of the oil to a large, lidded casserole pot over a medium-high heat. Add the shallot, smashed garlic cloves and ginger. Cook for 5 minutes until they are slightly golden. Add the chicken (breast down), water, carrots and whole peppercorns with a pinch of salt. Bring the water to the boil and reduce to a simmer, removing any scum that forms on the surface. After 25 minutes, carefully turn the chicken over and cover the pan with the lid. Simmer gently for a further 20 minutes or until the juices of the chicken run clear when piercing the meat.

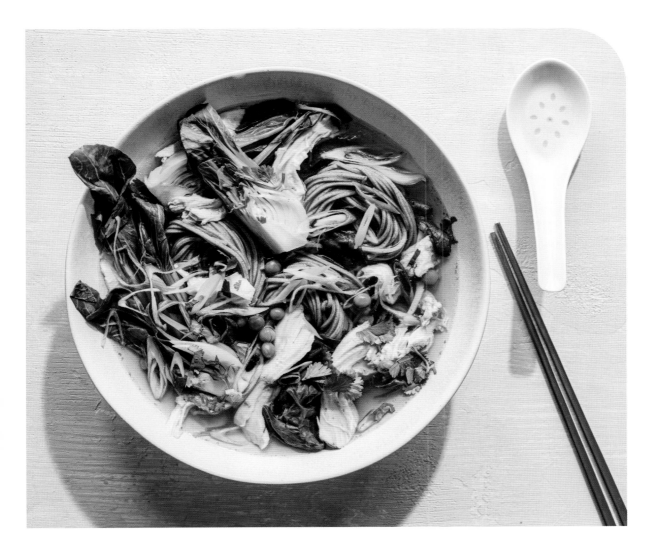

2. Once cooked, remove the chicken and leave it to rest for 10 minutes before shredding. To shred, tear the chicken off the bone (you can use your hands here!), removing any skin or fat, then use a fork to shred the meat.

3. Sieve the remaining liquid, discarding the vegetables, and return to the heat. Add the miso paste, spinach and chicken and stir through. Cook for 5 minutes on a low-medium heat. Season to taste.

4. Meanwhile, make the topping. Add the oil to a medium frying pan over a medium-high heat.

Add the garlic and chilli and cook for 2 minutes. Add the vegetables and cook for a further 5–10 minutes until cooked through.

5. Cook the noodles according to the packet instructions and drain. Divide the noodles between four deep bowls and top with the chicken soup, mixed veg, coriander and a squeeze of lime juice.

Store any leftovers in the fridge for up to 3 days.

kimchi grain bowl

When you fancy a spice hit, plus a WHOPPER of a hit on the variety counter. Lisa x

20 minutes | Serves 4
(if using pre-cooked rice and quinoa)

 7g per portion

 15 *(if using TGS kimchi)*

 kimchi

allergens: *sesame, soya*

2 tbsp tamari or light soy sauce

250g (7 oz) firm tofu, sliced

1 tbsp sesame oil or light olive oil

2 garlic cloves, sliced

2.5cm (1-in) piece of fresh ginger, peeled and grated

160g (2¾ oz) kale

250g (5¾ oz) pre-cooked brown rice

250g (4¼ oz) pre-cooked quinoa

TOPPING

200g (5½ oz) kimchi *(homemade, see page 260, or shop-bought)*

½ bunch spring onions, sliced

1 tbsp sesame seeds

squeeze of lime juice

 Fibre – add a small tin of canned sweetcorn to the kale
Variety – top with mixed beansprouts
Ferments – fermented hot sauce *(see page 227)*

1. Put half the tamari in a bowl, add the tofu and coat evenly.

2. Heat a frying pan over a medium-high heat and add the oil. Add the tofu slices and cook on each side for 2–3 minutes until golden. Reduce the heat to medium, add the garlic and ginger and cook for 1 minute. Remove the tofu from the pan and set aside.

3. Add the kale to the pan with the remaining tamari and cook for 2–4 minutes until the kale has wilted.

4. Heat the rice and quinoa according to the packet instructions and divide between two bowls.

5. Top the rice and quinoa with the tofu, kimchi, kale and spring onions and sprinkle over the sesame seeds. Add the lime juice and serve immediately.

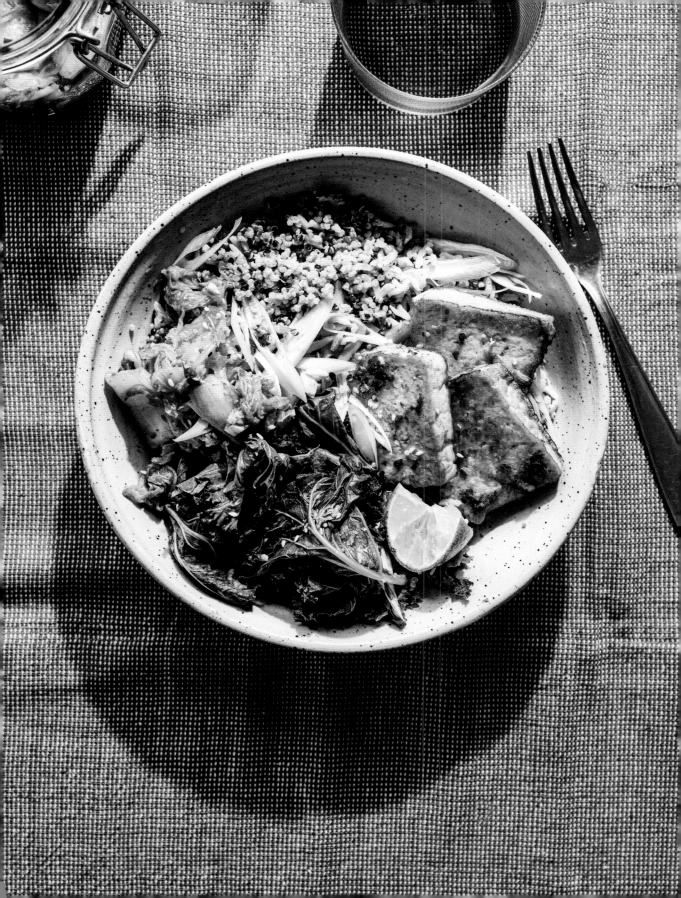

kim-cheese

Quick, high-variety, extremely addictive! Double whammy on the ferment front! Alana x

5 minutes | Serves 2

 6.7g per portion

 11 with TGS kimchi

 kimchi and sourdough

handful of fresh coriander

2 slices of sourdough
(*homemade, see page 252,
or shop-bought*)

60g (2¼ oz) goat's cheese

40g (1½ oz) watercress

100g (3½ oz) kimchi (*homemade, see page 260, or
shop-bought*)

allergens: *gluten, goat's milk*

1. Roughly chop the coriander and toast the sourdough.

2. Crumble the goat's cheese and roughly spread over the toast using the back of a fork. Top with the watercress, kimchi and coriander.

Best served and eaten immediately.

 Fibre – top with 2 tbsp crunchy seed and nut topping (*see page 229*)
Variety – top with a handful of rocket

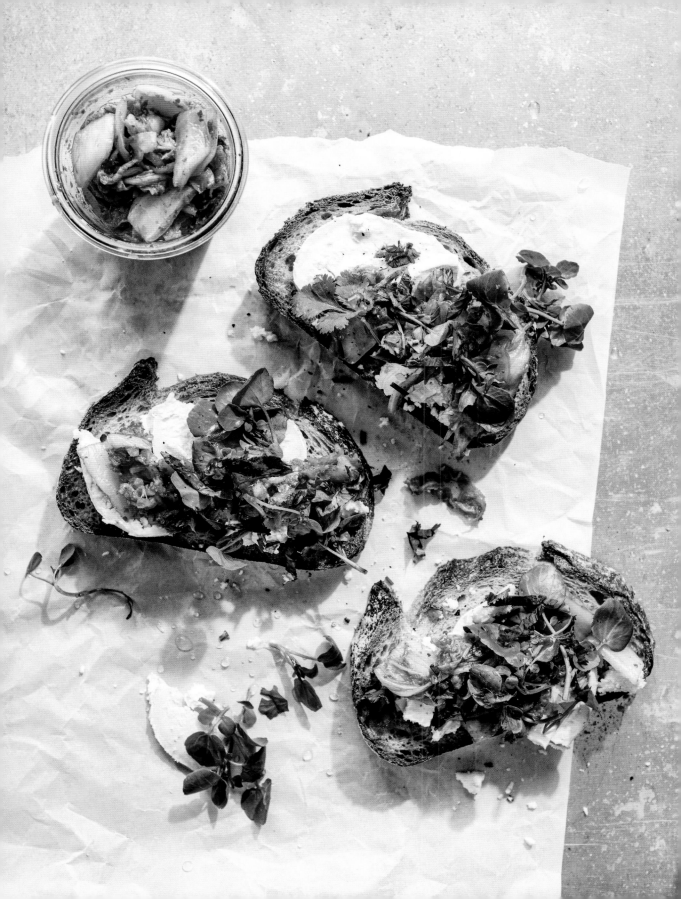

tomato and chickpea soup

There's something so comforting about a tomato soup. I like mine extra smookkeeey. Lisa x

1 hour | Serves 4

11g per portion

minimum 11

sourdough

allergens: *sesame (if adding fibre cracker), celery, gluten*

200g (7 oz) cherry or plum tomatoes, halved

3 tbsp olive oil

1 tbsp balsamic vinegar

1 leek, sliced

1 carrot *(skin on)*, finely diced

2 celery sticks, sliced

2 garlic cloves, crushed or grated

1 tsp paprika

1 tsp chilli flakes

1 x 400g (14-oz) can of chopped tomatoes

400ml (14 fl oz) vegetable stock

1 x 400g (14-oz) can of chickpeas, drained and rinsed

2 bay leaves

squeeze of lemon juice

200g (7 oz) greens, such as Savoy cabbage, cavolo nero or kale, leaves roughly shredded

1 tsp smoked paprika

salt and pepper

toasted sourdough *(homemade, see page 252, or shop-bought)*, to serve

Fibre and variety –
crumbled fibre crackers *(see page 157)*
Ferments – spoonful of milk kefir yogurt
(see page 264)

1. Preheat the oven to 180°C fan/200°C/400°F/gas mark 6.

2. Spread the tomatoes over a baking tray and drizzle with 1 tablespoon of the olive oil and balsamic vinegar. Season with salt and pepper and cook for 15–20 minutes.

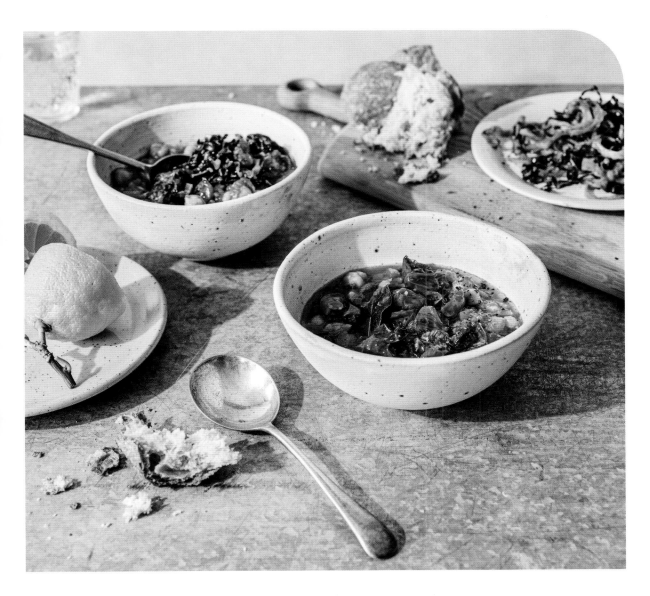

3. Heat 1 tbsp of the olive oil in a large pan over a medium heat. Add the leek, carrot and celery and cook for 5–10 minutes until softened, stirring occasionally. Add the garlic and cook for 2 minutes. Stir in the paprika and chilli flakes and cook for 1 minute. Add the canned tomatoes, vegetable stock, chickpeas and bay leaves. Partially cover with a lid, reduce the heat to a simmer and cook for about 20 minutes until slightly thickened. Stir in the roasted balsamic tomatoes and lemon juice. Season to taste and remove the bay leaves.

4. In a separate pan, add the remaining 1 teaspoon of olive oil over a medium heat. Add the greens and smoked paprika and stir-fry for 5 minutes until tender.

5. Serve the soup topped with the paprika greens and a side of toasted sourdough.

Any leftover soup can be stored in the fridge for up to 4 days or frozen for up to 1 month.

the
classics

spaghetti bolognese

Sometimes I take the additions in my bolognese a bit too far, ha! But always lentils for more fibre, then olives to jazz it up... Plus there's always the option to have mushrooms instead of beef?! Lisa x

1 hour | Serves 4+

11g with beef, 12g with mushrooms per portion

minimum 9

olives

allergens: *celery, cow's milk, gluten*

1–2 tbsp olive oil

1 onion, finely diced

2 carrots *(skin on)*, finely diced

2 celery sticks, finely diced

2 garlic cloves, crushed or grated

400g (14 oz) minced beef or mixed mushrooms, roughly chopped

1 x 400g (14-oz) can of chopped tomatoes

1 tbsp dried oregano

1 tbsp dried thyme

90g (3¼ oz) stoned olives *(optional)*, roughly chopped

200ml (7 fl oz) beef or vegetable stock

1 x 400g (14-oz) can of lentils green or puy, rinsed and drained

1 tbsp tomato purée

300g (10½ oz) spaghetti handful of fresh basil leaves, torn

60g (2¼ oz) Parmesan cheese, grated

salt and pepper

1. Add the olive oil to a large non-stick pan over a medium-high heat. Add the onion, carrots and celery, season with salt and cook for 5–10 minutes until softened. Add the garlic, cook for a minute, then add the minced beef or mixed mushrooms and cook for 10 minutes, stirring, until browned.

2. Add the oregano, thyme and olives and cook for 2 minutes. Add the canned tomatoes, stock and lentils and tomato purée then bring to the boil. Reduce to a simmer and cook for 40–50 minutes or until the sauce has thickened. Season to taste.

3. Bring a medium saucepan of salted water to the boil and cook the spaghetti according to the packet instructions.

4. To serve, mix together the spaghetti and the bolognese sauce, divide between bowls and top with the torn basil leaves and grated Parmesan. Store any leftovers in the fridge for up to 3 days or freeze the bolognese sauce for up to a month. Defrost thoroughly before reheating.

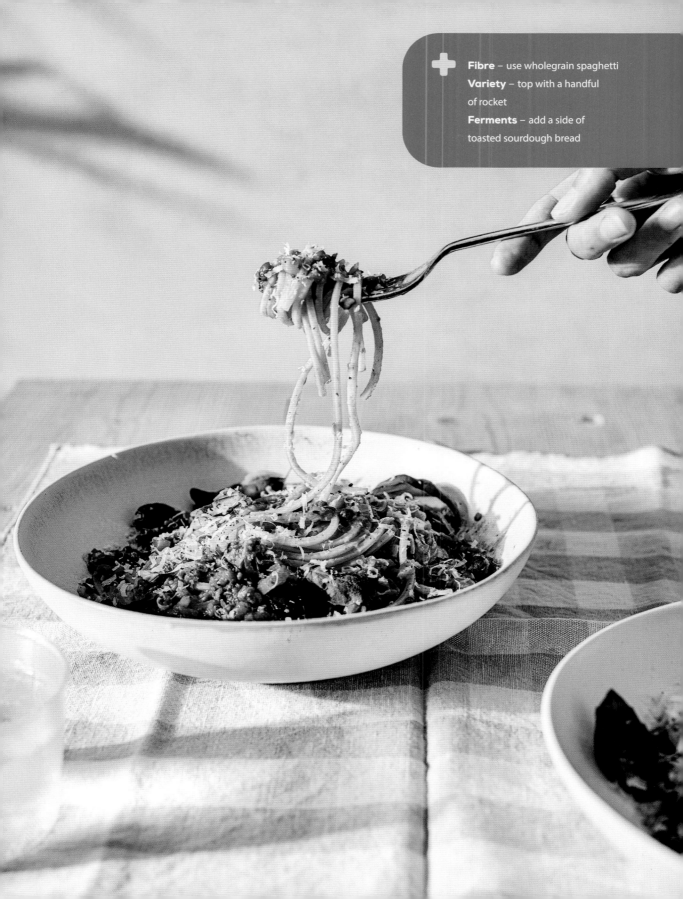

Fibre – use wholegrain spaghetti
Variety – top with a handful
of rocket
Ferments – add a side of
toasted sourdough bread

beetroot burgers with root vegetable chips

A wonderfully bright and light plant-based alternative. Alana x

1 hour | Serves 4+

minimum 13g per portion

minimum 8

milk kefir
yogurt, kimchi
or sauerkraut

allergens: *gluten, egg,
cow's milk, sesame*

BEETROOT BURGERS

1 tbsp olive oil, plus extra for
    brushing the burgers

1 red onion, finely chopped

2 tsp ground cumin

1 slice day-old sourdough

400g (14 oz) raw beetroot,
    coarsely grated

2 x 400g (14-oz) cans of
    chickpeas, drained and
    rinsed

2 heaped tbsp flaxseed

2 tbsp milk kefir yogurt
    *(homemade, see page 264,
    or shop-bought)*

1 egg

1 tbsp tahini

1 tbsp rice flour, plus extra
    if needed

salt and pepper

ROOT VEGETABLE CHIPS

1 large, sweet potato, *(skin
    on)* and sliced into chips

½ celeriac, peeled and sliced
    into chips

olive oil

TO SERVE *(optional)*

wholegrain buns

rocket

onion *(any variety)*, sliced

ferments, such as kimchi or
    sauerkraut *(homemade
    see pages 260 and 256,
    or shop-bought)*

1. Preheat the oven to 220°C/200°C fan/425°F/ gas mark 7 and line two medium baking trays with baking paper. Put the sweet potato and celeriac on one of the baking trays, drizzle with olive oil, season and set aside.

2. In a frying pan, heat 1 tablespoon of olive oil and fry the onion for 3–5 minutes until softened. Add the cumin and cook together for 1 minute.

Recipe continued overleaf

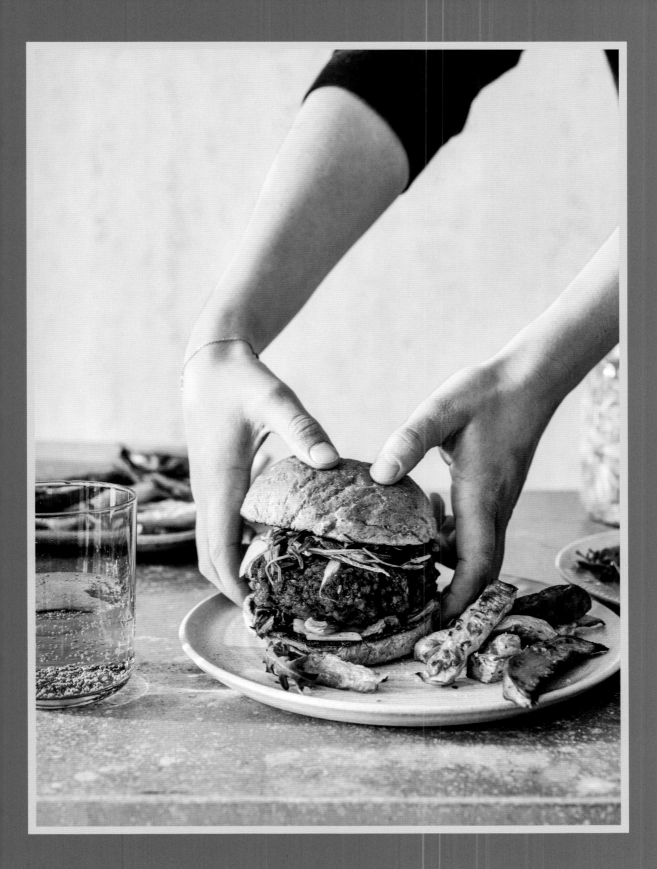

3. Put the sourdough in a food processor and pulse to breadcrumbs, then add the onion mixture along with the grated beetroot, chickpeas, flaxseed, milk kefir yogurt, egg, tahini and rice flour. Mix to a rough paste, then scrape into a bowl and season well. If the mixture is sticky, add a little more flour.

4. With damp hands, shape the mixture into about six burgers and space apart on the remaining baking tray. Brush the burgers with a little olive oil and bake in the oven alongside the root vegetable chips for 35–40 minutes until crisp and hot through.

5. Serve the burgers in wholegrain buns with rocket, onion and ferments as you wish.

Leftover beetroot burgers can be stored in an airtight container in the fridge for up to 4 days.

 Fibre – serve with sliced tomatoes
Variety – *a handful of rocket*
Ferments – fermented tomato ketchup or fermented hot sauce *(see pages 226 and 227)*

chicken nuggets

Nuggets are my go-to hangover food – we've added some flaxseed for a fibre boost so your gut bugs can have a post-party munch too. Lisa x

30 minutes | 2 as a main or 4 as a side

 5.6 g per portion

3

allergens: *nuts (almonds), eggs*

2 skinless chicken breasts

40g (1¾ oz) ground almonds

1 tsp paprika

2 tbsp ground flaxseed

1 egg

salt and pepper

1. Preheat the oven to 200°C/180°C fan/400°F/ gas mark 6 and line a medium baking tray with baking paper.

2. Using a sharp knife, cut the chicken into chunks. Mix the almonds, flaxseed and paprika in a shallow bowl and season well. In another shallow bowl, whisk the egg.

3. Coat the chicken chunks in the beaten egg and then the almond mixture one by one. Transfer to the lined baking tray and bake for 15–25 minutes until cooked through and slightly golden, turning halfway through cooking.

Best served immediately but any leftovers can be stored in the fridge for up to a day.

 Fibre and Variety – serve with a side of kefir tzatziki and sweet potato wedges *(see page 214)*
Ferments – fermented hot sauce or ketchup *(see pages 226 and 227)*

aubergine and sweet potato katsu curry

Anything with Katsu Curry in the title... SOLD! Alana x

40 minutes | Serves 4

 9.8g per portion

 minimum 11

 milk kefir yogurt

allergens: *nuts (almonds), eggs, soya (if using soy sauce), gluten*

100g (3½ oz) ground almonds

1 egg or 20ml (4 tsp) almond milk

1 aubergine, cut into 1cm (½-in) pieces

1 medium sweet potato (*skin on*), cut into 1cm (½-in) pieces

2 tbsp groundnut oil or a light olive oil

1 onion, diced

3 garlic cloves, crushed

2.5cm (1-in) piece of fresh ginger, peeled and grated

1 tbsp medium curry powder

1 tsp garam masala

½ tsp ground turmeric

2 carrots (*skin on*), grated

1 apple (*skin on*), grated

2 tbsp light soy sauce or tamari

1–2 tbsp tomato purée

500ml (18 fl oz) vegetable stock

salt and pepper

TO SERVE

240g wholegrain rice

handful fresh coriander

4 tbsp milk kefir yogurt

 Fibre and variety – corn salsa (*see page 225*)
Ferments – a side of kimchi or fermented hot sauce (*see pages 260 and 227*)

1. Preheat the oven to 180°C fan/200°C/400°F/ gas mark 6 and line two medium baking trays with baking paper. Put the ground almonds in a shallow bowl and season with salt and pepper. In another shallow bowl, whisk the egg or add the almond milk.

2. Coat the aubergine and sweet potato in the beaten egg or almond milk and then the almond mixture. Transfer to the lined baking trays and cook for 25–30 minutes until the vegetables are tender and the almond coating is golden.

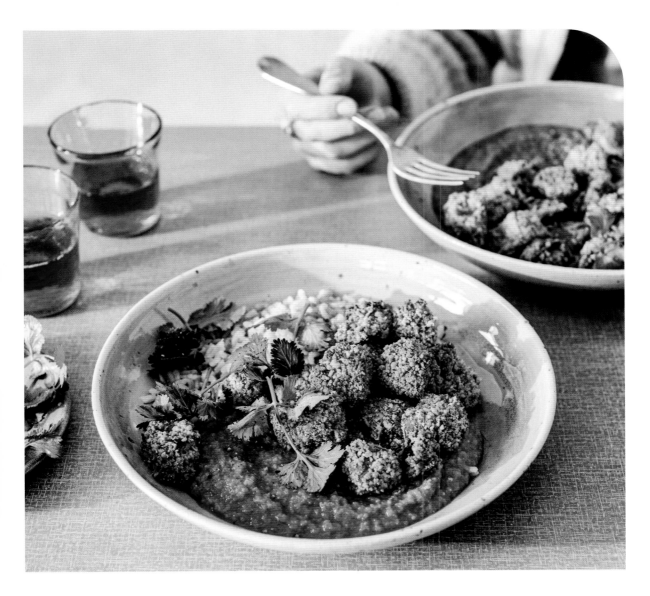

3. Meanwhile, cook the rice as per the packet instructions and set aside.

4. Heat the oil in a large pan over a medium-high heat. Add the onion and cook for 5–7 minutes until softened. Reduce the heat, add the garlic and ginger and cook for 2 minutes. Add all the spices and stir through. Add the carrot and apple and stir to combine. Add the soy sauce or tamari, tomato purée and stock. Increase the heat and bring to the boil, then reduce the heat and simmer for 20 minutes.

Remove from the heat and use a stick blender to blend to a smooth sauce. Season to taste.

5. To serve, divide the rice between four plates, add the sauce and top with the roast vegetables, fresh coriander and a dollop of milk kefir yogurt.

Store the sauce and vegetables in the fridge for up to 3 days. Rice should be stored for 1 day only and must be reheated until piping hot before eating.

sourdough pizza

WHAT A CROWD PLEASER. Get creative with toppings – I like to leave it to the guests if I'm entertaining as all sorts of tomfoolery and creativity ensues. Lisa x

30 minutes | Makes 2 pizzas

+ prep dough 1 day in advance

 see toppings

 see toppings

 sourdough

allergens: *gluten, milk, nuts (check per topping make dairy free using alternatives and omit the nuts if needed)*

PIZZA BASE
(MAKES TWO BASES)

1 tbsp olive oil, plus extra
  for greasing

275g (9¾ oz) strong white
  bread flour, plus extra
  for dusting

55g (2 oz) sourdough
  starter *(see page 252)*

185g (6½ oz) water

5g (⅛ oz) salt

TOPPINGS

TOMATO SAUCE

1 x 200g can of chopped
  tomatoes

salt and pepper

60g mozzarella, feta, goat's
  cheese *(or 30g Parmesan
  cheese)*

PLANT-BASED TOPPINGS

¼ x 400g (14-oz) can of
  chickpeas *(+2g fibre)*

handful of broccoli *(+2.8g fibre)*

5–6 asparagus spears *(+1.4g fibre)*

80g (2¾ oz) jarred Jerusalem
  artichokes *(+4g fibre)*

½ pepper, any colour *(+1.8g fibre)*

handful of chopped cooked
  aubergine *(+2.5g fibre)*

80g (2¾ oz) tomatoes *(+0.9g fibre)*

80g (2¾ oz) mushrooms
  (+0.8g fibre)

TOPPINGS TO ADD
ONCE COOKED

handful of rocket or spinach

1 tsp chilli flakes

50g jarred sun-dried
  tomatoes

1 tbsp crunchy seed and nut
  mix *(see page 229)*

50g sauerkraut *(homemade,
  see page 256, or shop-bought)*

drizzle of milk kefir yogurt
  *(homemade, see page 264,
  or shop-bought)*

drizzle of fermented hot
  sauce *(homemade, see
  page 227, or shop-bought)*

side of fermented tomato
  ketchup *(homemade, see
  page 226, or shop-bought)*

handful of fresh basil leaves,
  torn

2 tbsp walnut pesto
  (homemade, see page 231)

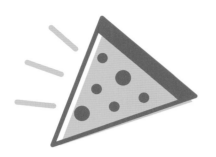

Jarred vegetables are great to have in the pantry to add on... think artichokes, peppers, sun-dried tomatoes and olives, etc. Also we prep the dough the day before, so you can spend your time chattin', not rollin' and kneadin'.

1. To make the pizza bases, add all the ingredients to an oiled bowl and use your fingers to mix until you have a sticky dough ball. Cover with a tea towel and leave to sit for 30 minutes at room temperature. After 30 minutes turn the dough out onto a work surface and use the 'slap and fold' method to stretch and fold the dough until it feels stronger, smoother and more elastic. This can take around 10 minutes – keep going! Use a dough scraper to mould the dough into a ball. Return to the bowl, cover again and leave to sit at room temperature for 6 hours until the dough has begun to show signs of fermentation.

2. After 6 hours, turn the dough out onto a work surface, adding a dusting of flour if required, and use scales to portion into two equal balls. Place the dough balls on a lightly floured baking tray with high sides and cover with oiled clingfilm. Put in the fridge for 12–24 hours until ready to cook. (The dough will need to be brought to room temperature before cooking, so remove from the fridge for 30–60 minutes beforehand.)

3. Preheat the oven to 220°C fan/240°C/475°F/gas mark 9. Prep all your toppings. To prep the tomato sauce, add the chopped tomatoes to a bowl and season with salt and pepper.

4. To shape the dough, dust a work surface with flour and delicately work and stretch the dough into a round base roughly 25–27cm (10–12 in) in diameter.

5. Place a non-stick frying pan (the same size as your pizza base) over a high heat. Once the pan is hot, carefully add the dough. Next, add the tomato sauce, spreading it with the back of a spoon, then quickly arrange the toppings. Cook over a high heat for 2–4 minutes until the base has turned golden. Then use a spatula to remove from the pan and transfer to a baking tray. Bake in the oven for 8 minutes. Repeat with the second base. Finish by adding any of the extra toppings once cooked.

Leftovers will keep in the fridge for up to a day.

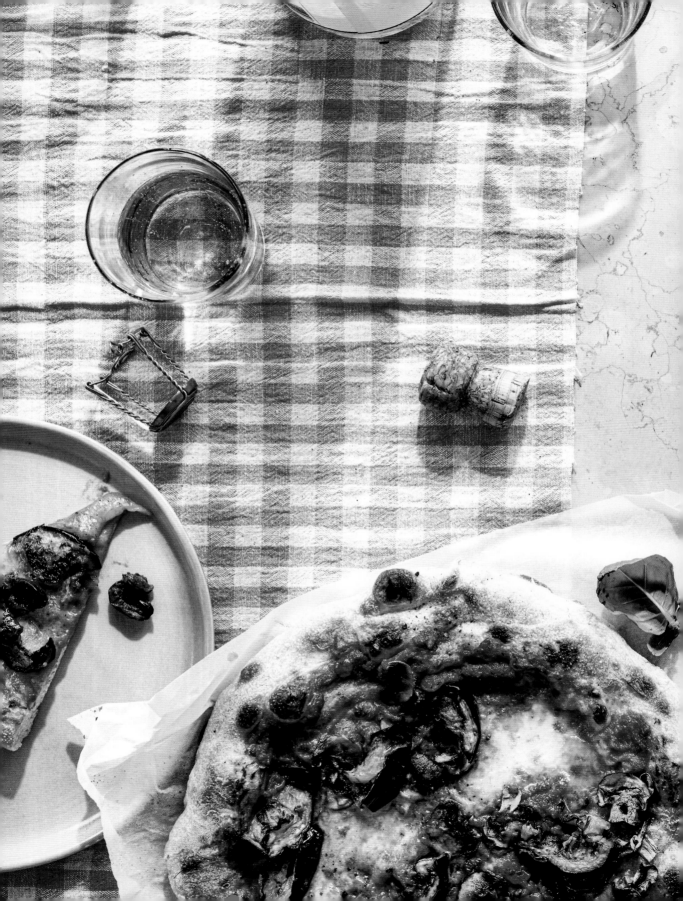

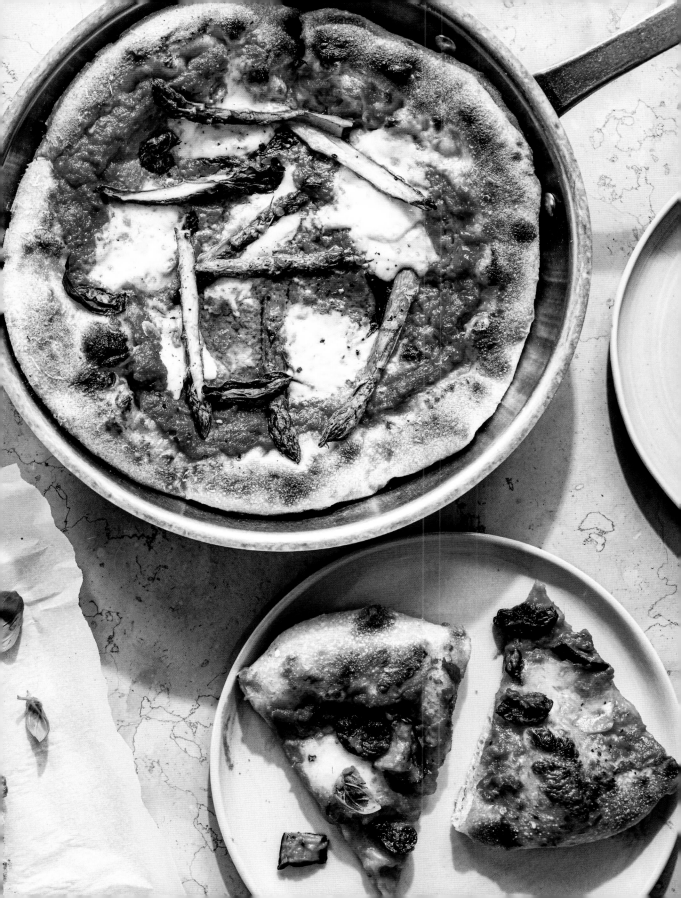

veggie chilli

Speaks for itself. We love to pour the leftovers onto baked sweet potatoes or our loaded fries, and would highly recommend with a dollop of kefir ;) Alana x

50 minutes | Serves 4–6

12g per portion

minimum 10

allergens: *check stock cubes for allergens*

2 tbsp olive oil

1 onion, diced

1 pepper *(any colour)*, cored, deseeded and sliced

2 garlic cloves, crushed

1 red chilli, deseeded and finely chopped

2 tsp paprika

2 tsp ground cumin

½–1 tsp hot chilli powder

1 medium butternut squash *(skin on)*, cut into 2.5cm (1-in) cubes

1 x 400g (14-oz) can of chopped tomatoes

300ml (10 fl oz) vegetable stock

1 x 400g (14-oz) can of red kidney beans, drained and rinsed

300g (10½ oz) wholegrain rice

1 lime, quartered

salt and pepper

Fibre – use wholegrain rice instead of white rice

Variety – top with a handful of chopped fresh coriander

Ferments – a spoonful of milk kefir yogurt *(homemade, see page 264)*

1. Add the olive oil to a large non-stick pan over a medium-high heat. Add the onion, season and cook for 5–10 minutes until softened. Add the pepper, garlic and chilli and cook for 2 minutes. Add the squash and stir to coat in the spices.

2. Pour in the tomatoes, swill a splash of water around the can and add this too along with the stock.

Bring to the boil, reduce to a simmer, tip in the kidney beans and cook for 20–30 minutes until the squash is tender. Season to taste.

3. Meanwhile, cook the rice according to the packet instructions.

4. Serve the vegetable chilli with the rice and a squeeze of fresh lime juice.

Store any leftover chilli in the fridge for up to 4 days or freeze for up to a month.

one-pot butter bean, broccoli and leeks

A simple week-night dinner; fresh, quick and ooh so comforting. Lisa x

30 minutes | Serves 2

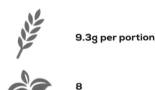

9.3g per portion

8

allergens: *cow's milk*

1 tbsp butter

1 leek

200g (7 oz) broccoli *(florets and stalks),* roughly chopped

3 sprigs of thyme

2 garlic cloves, crushed

1 tbsp capers, finely chopped

1 x 400g (14-oz) can of butter beans, drained and rinsed

1 bay leaf

handful of fresh flat-leaf parsley, finely chopped

½ mozzarella ball, torn

salt and pepper

1. Melt the butter in a medium pan over a medium-high heat. Add the leek, cut-side down, to soak up the butter. Season and cook for 2–4 minutes until golden, reducing the heat if the leeks begin to catch.

2. Add the broccoli and season with salt and pepper. Stir in the thyme sprigs, garlic and capers. Add 200ml (7 fl oz) water, followed by the butter beans, bay leaf and parsley.

3. Cover with a lid, reduce the heat and simmer gently for 20 minutes. When cooked, remove the bay leaf and thyme sprigs and season to taste.

4. To serve, divide between two bowls and top with the torn mozzarella and freshly ground black pepper.

Store any leftovers in the fridge for up to 2 days.

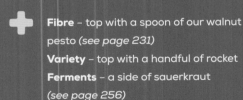

Fibre – top with a spoon of our walnut pesto *(see page 231)*

Variety – top with a handful of rocket

Ferments – a side of sauerkraut *(see page 256)*

baked salmon topped with sourdough crumbs

Fuss-free – great with a veg tray bake bonanza. Lisa x

30 minutes | Serves 2

 6.1g

 minimum 6

 olives and sourdough

1 slice of day-old sourdough *(homemade, see page 252, or shop-bought)*

1½ tbsp olive oil

1 lemon, quartered

1 fennel bulb, finely sliced

1 red onion, sliced

2 handfuls of cherry tomatoes

100g jarred artichoke, drained

2 salmon fillets

2 garlic cloves, finely sliced

handful of stoned black olives

handful of fresh herbs, such as basil or flat-leaf parsley, roughly chopped

salt and pepper

allergens: *gluten, fish, celery, nuts (walnuts, if adding walnut pesto)*

1. Preheat the oven to 180°C fan/200°C/400°F/gas mark 6 and line a baking tray with baking paper. Add the sourdough to a blender and pulse to breadcrumbs, then stir in the ½ tablespoon of olive oil. Season the salmon with salt and pepper and a squeeze of lemon juice.

2. Place the fennel, onion, tomatoes and jarred artichokes in a mixing bowl, season well and coat with the remaining olive oil. Spread out over a medium baking tray and cook for 15 minutes.

3. Remove the tray from the oven, stir in the garlic and olives, add the salmon and cover the salmon and vegetables with the sourdough breadcrumbs.

Return to the oven and cook for a further 15–20 minutes until the salmon is cooked through.

4. Serve garnished with the chopped fresh herbs and an extra squeeze of lemon juice.

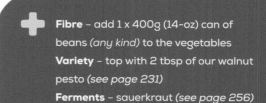

Fibre – add 1 x 400g (14-oz) can of beans *(any kind)* to the vegetables
Variety – top with 2 tbsp of our walnut pesto *(see page 231)*
Ferments – sauerkraut *(see page 256)*

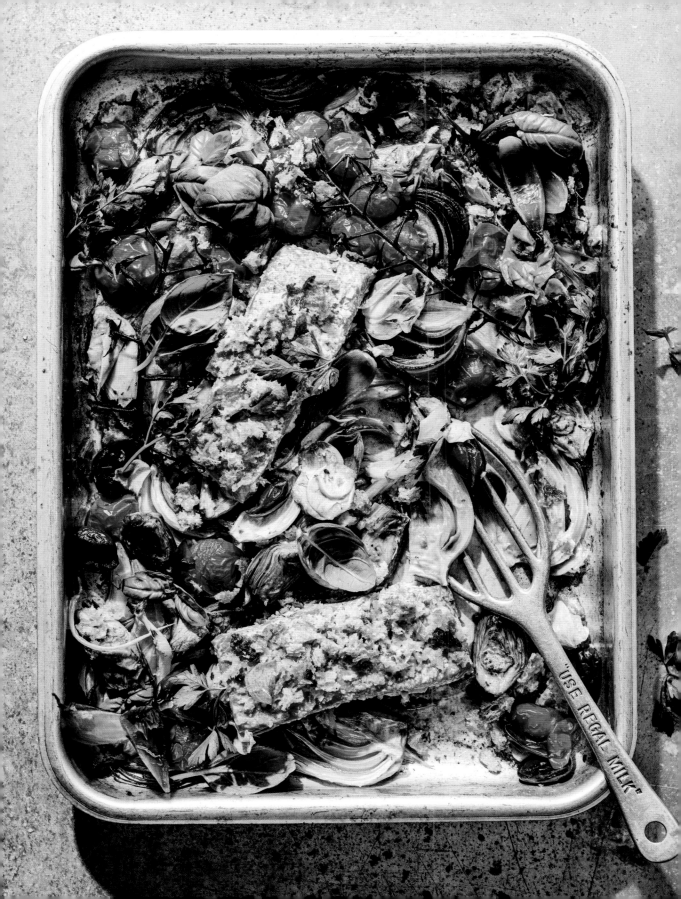

aubergine parmigiana with spicy courgettes

Homemade, bubbly, cheesy – all the good stuff. Lisa x

1 hour 10 minutes | Serves 4

9.8g per portion

minimum 9

allergens: *cow's milk*

2 large aubergines, cut into
    1cm- (½-in-) thick slices

1 tbsp olive oil

TOMATO SAUCE

1 tbsp olive oil

1 onion (*brown or red*), diced

1 pepper (*red, yellow or
    sweet pointed*)

2 garlic cloves, smashed

1 tsp dried oregano

1 tsp dried thyme

pinch of chilli flakes

1 x 400g (14-oz) can of
    chopped tomatoes

1 x 250g (9-oz) packet
    cooked lentils (*green, Puy
    or beluga*)

125g (5½ oz) mozzarella

60g (2¼ oz) Parmesan
    cheese, finely grated

salt and pepper

SPICY COURGETTES

1 tbsp olive oil

2 courgettes, sliced

1 garlic clove, finely sliced

1 red chilli, deseeded and
    finely sliced

squeeze of lemon juice

1. Preheat the oven to 180°C fan/200°C/400°F/gas mark 6. Arrange the aubergine slices on one large or two medium baking trays, drizzle with olive oil and season. Cook for 15–20 minutes, then remove from the oven and set aside.

2. To make the tomato sauce, place the oil in a saucepan over a medium heat, add the onion and cook for 5–7 minutes until softened. Add the pepper, cook for 2 minutes, then add the garlic, oregano, thyme, chilli flakes and a pinch of salt. Add the canned tomatoes, swill a splash of water around the can and add this too. Bring the sauce to the boil, then reduce to a simmer for 25–30 minutes, stirring occasionally. Once reduced, use a stick blender to blend to a smooth sauce. Add the lentils, season and stir to combine.

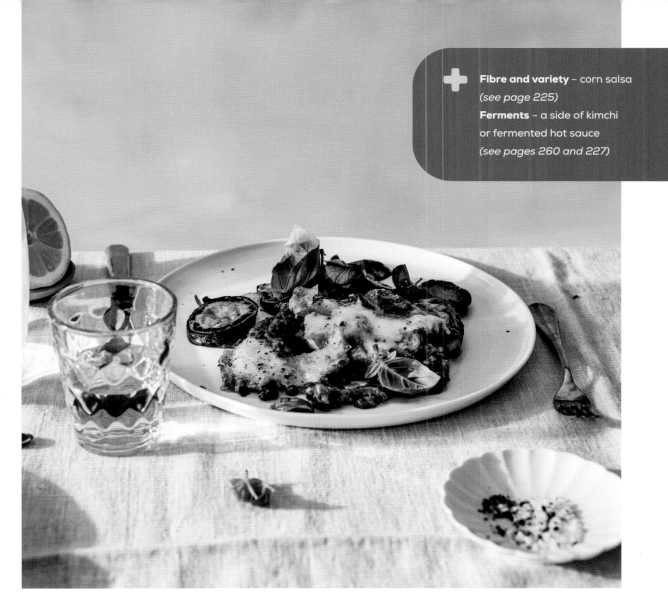

Fibre and variety – corn salsa
(see page 225)
Ferments – a side of kimchi
or fermented hot sauce
(see pages 260 and 227)

3. Add one-third of the tomato and lentil sauce to a medium baking dish, and spread over the base, followed by a single layer of half the aubergines. Repeat with one-third of the sauce and the remaining aubergines before finishing with the remaining tomato sauce on top. Roughly tear the mozzarella and scatter over the top along with the Parmesan. Bake for 35–40 minutes until bubbling.

4. For the spicy courgettes, place the olive oil in a non-stick pan over a medium-high heat. Add the garlic and chilli and cook for a minute before adding the courgettes. Cook for 2–3 minutes on each side until slightly golden. Add a squeeze of lemon juice before serving.

Best served immediately, but it can also be stored in the fridge for up to 3 days.

spiced bean and jackfruit tacos

I'll be honest, I had to be convinced on jackfruit – I was like WAH? But now I'm a convert, and this is great for having the guys and gals round for a booch/mocktail/margarita! Alana x

40 minutes | Serves 4

 17g

 minimum 12

 milk kefir yogurt

allergens: *gluten, cow's milk*

SPICED BEAN AND JACKFRUIT FILLING

- **1–2 tbsp** olive oil
- **1** small red onion, sliced
- **1** pepper, cored, deseeded and sliced
- **1** large garlic clove, crushed
- **2 tsp** ground cumin
- **2 tsp** smoked paprika
- **1 tsp** chilli flakes *(optional)*
- **1 x** 400g (14-oz) can of jackfruit, drained
- **1 x** 400g (14-oz) can of black beans, drained and rinsed
- **3 tbsp** tomato purée
- salt and pepper
- **squeeze** of lime juice

SMASHED AVOCADO

- **1** avocado, peeled and stoned
- **1** shallot, diced
- **squeeze** of lime juice
- **1 tsp** chilli flakes *(optional)*

TO SERVE

- milk kefir yogurt *(homemade, see page 264, or shop-bought)*
- **4–8** small wholemeal wraps
- **2 handfuls** of fresh coriander, roughly chopped
- **1** lime, cut into wedges

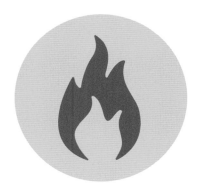

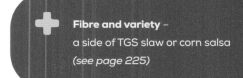

✚ **Fibre and variety** –
a side of TGS slaw or corn salsa
(*see page 225*)

1. Preheat the oven to 180°C fan/200°C/400°F/gas mark 6.

2. Place the oil in a medium saucepan, add the onion and cook for 5–7 minutes until softened. Add the pepper, cook for 2 minutes, then add the garlic, cumin, paprika, chilli flakes and a good pinch of salt. Add the canned jackfruit, black beans and tomato purée, together with 200ml (3½ fl oz) water. Bring the sauce to the boil, then reduce the heat and simmer for 25–30 minutes, stirring occasionally. Once the jackfruit has softened, use a fork to break it apart. Add a squeeze of lime juice and cook for a further 5 minutes. If the mixture looks a little dry, add a splash of water.

3. To make the smashed avocado, add the avocado to a bowl and mash with a fork to your desired consistency. Add the shallot, lime juice and chilli flakes, if using, and mix. Season to taste.

4. Add the wraps to the oven for the final 2 minutes of cooking to warm through.

5. To serve, spread a spoon of milk kefir yogurt over the warm wraps, top with some jackfruit and bean filling, smashed avocado and slaw or corn salsa, if you like.

TACO SALAD

Smashed avocado is best eaten fresh. Store any leftover corn salsa and jackfruit and black bean filling in the fridge for up to 3 days. Add to a bed of mixed leaves and fresh smashed avocado for a taco-style salad.

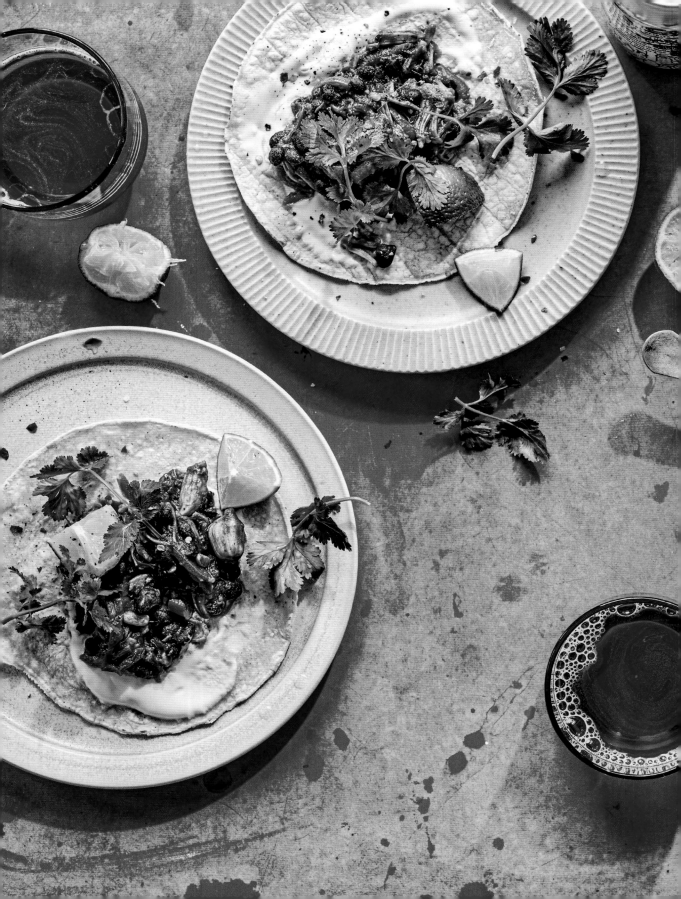

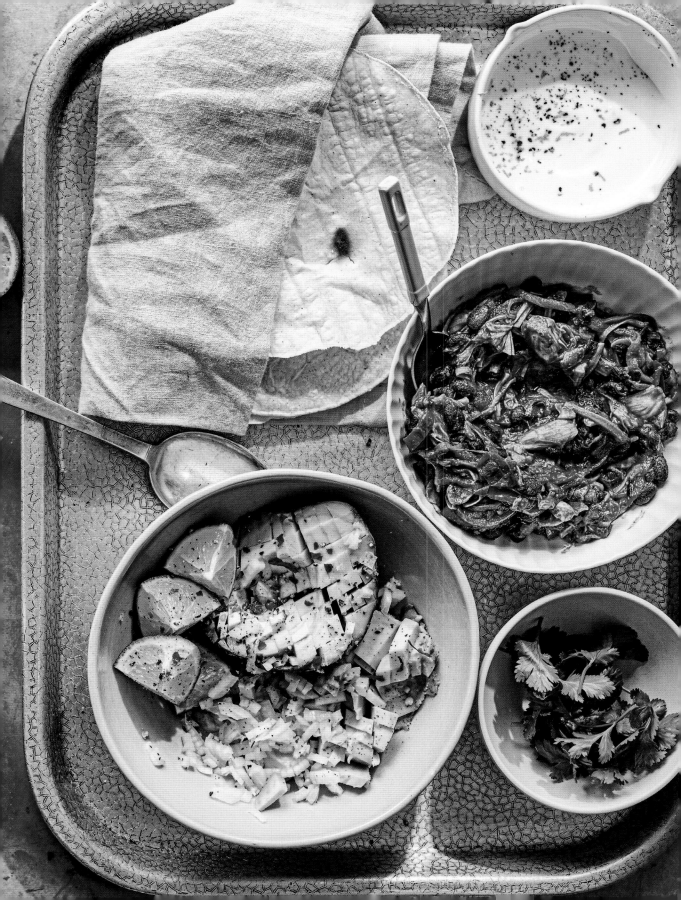

pantry fishcakes with celeriac slaw

Lauren on our team originally made this after a cupboard raid when it was snowing and she couldn't get to the shops! A budget week-night dinner when your food stores are running low; keep a couple of tins of fish in the pantry, in case you're caught short in extreme weather conditions like Lauren. x

1 hour | Makes 6 fish cakes, serves 2–3

 8.7g per portion

 minimum 6

 milk kefir yogurt

allergens: *fish, eggs, cow's milk, celery*

1 medium potato (*skin on*), cut into 2.5cm (1-in) chunks

1 medium sweet potato (*skin on*), cut into 2.5cm (1-in) chunks

2 x 100g (3½-oz) cans of salmon or mackerel, drained

4 spring onions, sliced into rounds

2 handfuls of fresh flat-leaf parsley, chopped

1 egg, beaten

zest and juice of ½ lemon

CELERIAC SLAW

½ celeriac, peeled

4 tbsp milk kefir yogurt (*homemade, see page 264, or shop-bought*)

salt and pepper

 Fibre – a side of hummus (*see page 216*)
Variety – top the fish cakes with a handful of watercress
Ferments – a side of sauerkraut (*see page 256*)

1. Preheat the oven to 180°C fan/200°C/400°F/gas mark 6 and line a baking tray with baking paper.

2. Bring a medium saucepan of salted water to the boil. Add both potatoes and cook for 20–25 minutes until tender. Remove from the heat, drain and steam-dry for 5 minutes. Roughly mash using a potato masher.

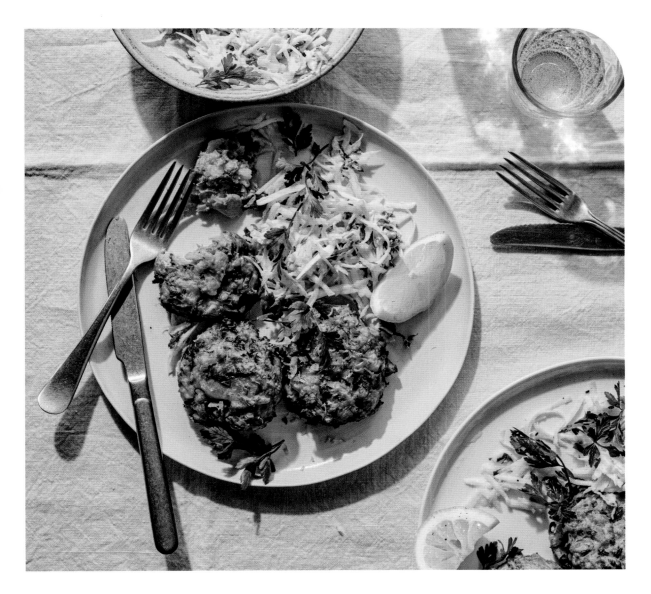

3. Transfer the mashed potato to a medium mixing bowl, add the salmon or mackerel, spring onions, half the parsley and the beaten egg. Mix to combine and season well before stirring in the lemon zest and a squeeze of juice. Using your hands, mould the mixture into 6 fishcakes and transfer to the lined baking tray. Bake for 30–35 minutes until golden, turning halfway through cooking.

4. While the fishcakes are in the oven, grate the celeriac and add to a bowl. Mix in the milk kefir yogurt, remaining parsley and a squeeze of lemon juice. Season to taste.

5. Serve the fishcakes alongside the celeriac slaw.

Any leftover fishcakes and slaw can be stored in the fridge for up to 2 days.

loaded fries

Great for the members of the household who love a kebab/chippie, a crowd pleaser for all the family/roommates! Alana x

40 minutes | Serves 2+

13g per portion

minimum 11

milk kefir yogurt

allergens: *cow's milk*

FRIES

2–3 root vegetables (*skin on*), such as sweet potato, potato, parsnip, small celeriac, carrots, cut into chunky chips

1 tsp garlic powder

1 tsp smoked paprika

1–2 tbsp olive oil

TOPPINGS

2 portions of veggie chilli (*see page 188*)

60g (2¼ oz) feta cheese, crumbled

2 tbsp milk kefir yogurt (*homemade, see page 264, or shop-bought*) or kefir tzatziki (*see page 214*)

handful of fresh coriander, chopped

squeeze of lime juice

---

1. Preheat the oven to 180°C fan/ 200°C/400°F/ gas mark 6 and line a medium baking tray with baking paper.

2. Bring a pan of salted water to the boil, add the root vegetables and parboil for 5–7 minutes. Drain and leave to steam-dry for 2 minutes.

3. Scatter the vegetables over the lined tray, add the garlic powder, smoked paprika and olive oil. Combine to coat and season well. Cook for 30 minutes until golden brown, stirring after 20 minutes.

4. Serve the fries topped with chilli, feta, a dollop of milk kefir yogurt, fresh coriander and a squeeze of lime juice.

Store veggie chilli in the fridge for up to 4 days. Serve the chips straight away.

Fibre – top with sliced avocado
Variety – top with 2 tbsp crunchy seed and nut mix (*see page 229*)
Ferments – top with kimchi or fermented hot sauce (*see pages 260 and 227*)

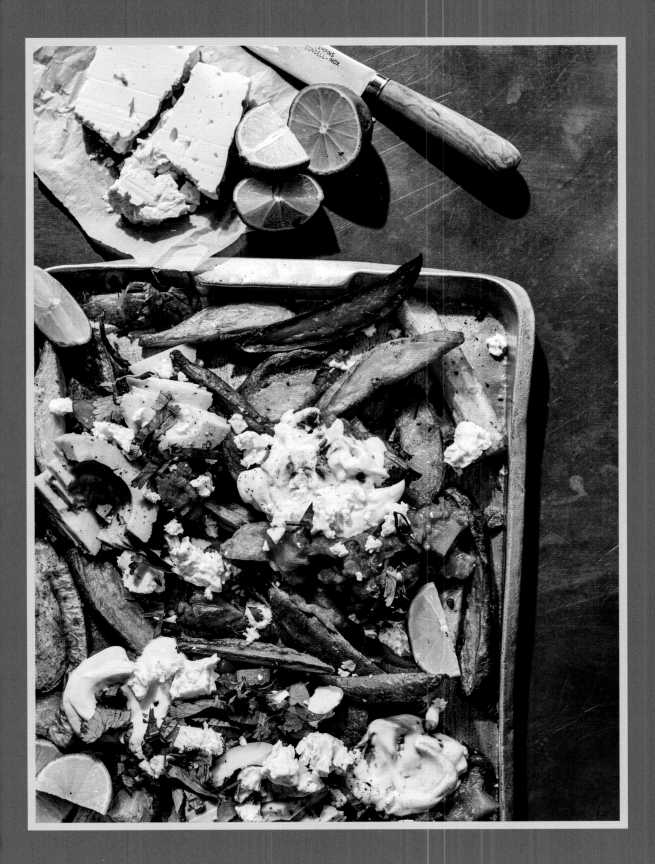

lentil shepherd's pie

You've got the family round on a Sunday – make this to please them and all your microbial relatives too. Trust us on the beetroot juice, but if you can't get hold of any, just use 200ml (7 fl oz) red wine. Alana x

1½ hours | Serves 4+

8.6g per portion

12

milk kefir yogurt

allergens: *cow's milk (if using milk kefir yogurt), gluten, fish (if using Worcestershire sauce), soya (if using Worcestershire sauce)*

- **1** large potato *(skin on)*, cut into cubes, cut into 2.5cm (1-in) chunks
- **1** medium sweet potato (skin on), cut into cubes
- **2 tbsp** milk kefir yogurt *(homemade, see page 264, or shop-bought – optional)*
- **2 tbsp** olive oil
- **1** leek, cut into rounds
- **2** carrots *(skin on)*, diced
- **2–3** garlic cloves, crushed
- **1 tbsp** dried thyme

- **1** small swede, peeled and cubed, cut into 2.5cm (1-in) chunks
- **1 x 400g (14-oz)** can of green lentils, drained and rinsed
- **200ml (7 fl oz)** pressed beetroot juice
- **1 x 400g (14-oz)** can of chopped tomatoes
- **200ml (7 fl oz)** vegetable stock
- **1 tbsp** tomato purée
- **1 tbsp** Worcestershire sauce (optional)
- salt and pepper

Fibre – a side of broccoli
Variety – 2 handfuls of frozen peas added to the pie mixture for the final 5 minutes of cooking
Ferments – side of fermented ketchup or hot sauce *(see pages 226 and 227)*

1. Preheat the oven to 200°C fan/220°C/425°F/gas mark 7.

2. Bring a large pan of salted water to the boil. Add the potatoes and cook for 20–25 minutes until tender. Once cooked, drain and use a potato masher to mash by hand. Once cool, add the kefir (if using) and season.

3. Add the olive oil to a large pan over a medium-high heat. Add the leek and carrots and season.

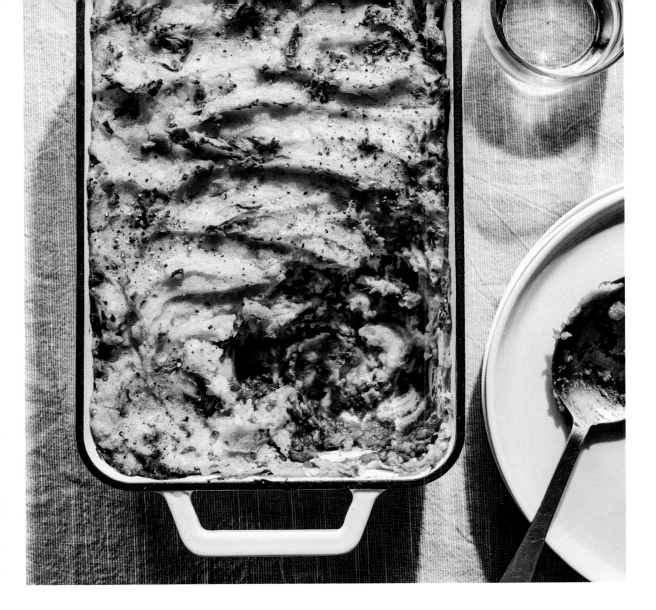

Cook for 5–10 minutes, stirring occasionally, until the vegetables begin to soften. Add the garlic and thyme and cook for 2 minutes. After this next, add the swede and lentils and stir to coat. Add the beetroot juice and leave to bubble for 1 minute before adding the canned tomatoes, vegetable stock and tomato purée. Season well with salt and pepper, bring to the boil, and then reduce the heat to a simmer and cook for 30–35 minutes until the sauce has thickened. Add the Worcestershire sauce for the final 5 minutes of cooking, if using.

4. Transfer the filling to an ovenproof baking dish. Top with the mashed potatoes and bake for 30–40 minutes until bubbling and crispy on top.

Store any leftovers in the fridge for up to 4 days.

mushroom and mixed bean hotpot

Cosy evening, glass of vino, tele on. Uhuh. Also, go crazy on the different mushroom types – lots of supermarkets do mixed boxes now. Lisa x

1½ hours | Serves 4

13g per portion

11

allergens: *celery, gluten (check shop-bought stock cubes)*

2 tbsp olive oil

1 onion, finely diced

1 carrot *(skin on)*, finely diced

2 celery sticks, finely diced

3 garlic cloves, crushed

500g (1 lb 2 oz) mushrooms *(any variety)*, roughly chopped

2 tsp dried rosemary

1 tbsp dried thyme

500ml (18 fl oz) mushroom or vegetable stock

1 x 400g (14-oz) can of black beans, drained and rinsed

1 x 400g (14-oz) can of cannellini beans, drained and rinsed

1 medium potato *(skin on)*, sliced into 5mm (¼-in) thick rounds

1 parsnip (skin on), sliced into 5mm (¼-in) thick rounds

salt and pepper

1. Preheat the oven to 180°C fan/200°C/400°F/gas mark 6.

2. Over a medium heat, add half the olive oil to a casserole dish. Add the onion, carrot and celery and cook for 5–10 minutes until softened. Add the garlic and cook for 2 minutes, stirring. Add the mushrooms, rosemary and thyme, season and cook, stirring, until browned.

3. Stir in the stock and the beans. Bring to the boil and then reduce to a simmer for 10–15 minutes. Meanwhile, bring a pan of salted water to the boil and parboil the potato and parsnip for 5 minutes.

4. Arrange the potato and parsnip on top of the mushroom mixture, brush with olive oil and season. Cook in the oven for 30–40 minutes until golden.

Store any leftovers in an airtight container in the fridge for up to 3 days.

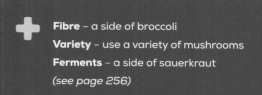

Fibre – a side of broccoli
Variety – use a variety of mushrooms
Ferments – a side of sauerkraut
(see page 256)

red lentil dahl

Bit of cauliflower love: it is a source of vitamin C, per portion gives 7% of recommended daily fibre. If you like a bit more spice, like me, add a tsp of chilli flakes. Lisa x

50 minutes | Serves 4

9.1 g per portion

13

milk kefir yogurt

allergens: *cow's milk, nuts (cashews)*

250g (9 oz) split red lentils

3 tbsp coconut oil

4 small or 1 medium shallot, finely diced

5cm (2-in) piece of fresh ginger, peeled and finely grated

2 garlic cloves, finely grated or crushed

1–2 tsp chilli flakes

1 tsp ground turmeric

2 tsp ground coriander

2 tsp ground cumin

500ml (18 fl oz) vegetable stock

1 x 400ml (14-fl oz) can of coconut milk

1 small cauliflower, broken into florets

2 carrots *(skin on)*, roughly chopped

2 tbsp tomato purée

1 lime

40g (1½ oz) cashews, roughly chopped

milk kefir yogurt *(homemade, see page 264, or shop-bought)*

2 handfuls of fresh coriander

salt and pepper

1. Preheat the oven to 180°C fan/200°C/400°F/gas mark 6. Use a sieve to rinse the red lentils until the water runs clear. Set aside.

2. Heat 1 tablespoon of the coconut oil in a large pan over a medium heat. Add the shallots and cook for 5–10 minutes until softened, stirring occasionally. Add the ginger, garlic and chilli flakes and cook for 2 minutes. Add the turmeric, 1 teaspoon of the ground cumin and ground coriander, then stir in the lentils and vegetable stock and cook for 5 minutes until the lentils begin to soak up the stock.

3. Add the coconut milk and tomato purée, bring to the boil, then reduce to a simmer, stirring occasionally. Cook until the lentils are cooked through (30 minutes).

Recipe continued overleaf

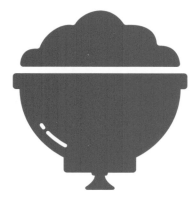

4. Melt the remaining coconut oil in a small saucepan and pour into a mixing bowl with the remaining spices. Add the cauliflower, carrots and a squeeze of lime juice, stir to coat and then season. Transfer to a medium baking tray and roast for 25–30 minutes until golden. Add the cashews for the final 5 minutes of cooking.

5. To serve, divide the dahl between four deep bowls and top with the roasted vegetables and cashews, fresh coriander and dollop of milk kefir yogurt.

Store any leftovers in the fridge for up to 3 days.

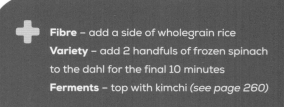

Fibre – add a side of wholegrain rice
Variety – add 2 handfuls of frozen spinach to the dahl for the final 10 minutes
Ferments – top with kimchi *(see page 260)*

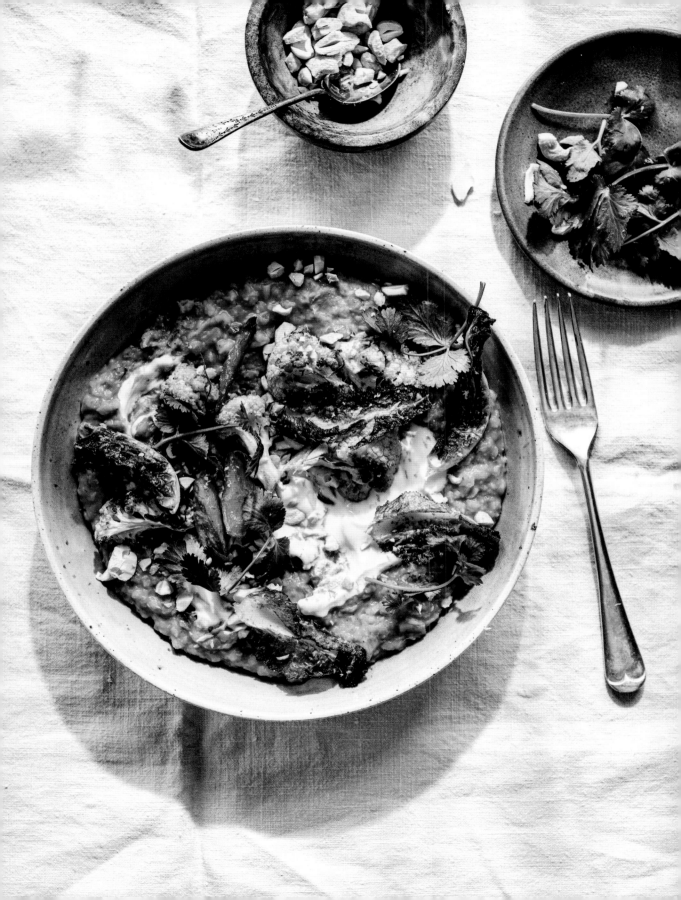

chickpea balls topped with tomato sauce and walnut pesto

These are also great as a tapas-style starter too... Alana x

1½ hours | Serves 2

15g per portion

minimum 9

sourdough

allergens: *cow's milk, gluten, nuts (walnuts), eggs*

2 tbsp olive oil

1 onion, finely diced

1 red pepper, deseeded and roughly chopped

1 x 400g (14-oz) can of chopped tomatoes

3 garlic cloves, smashed

1 tsp dried oregano

pinch of chilli flakes

1 slice of day-old sourdough *(homemade, see page 252, or shop-bought)*, roughly torn

1 x 400g (14-oz) can of chickpeas, drained and rinsed

50g (1¾ oz) sun-dried tomatoes

¼ bunch of fresh basil, leaves only

1 egg

salt and pepper

TO SERVE

pesto *(homemade, see page 231, or shop-bought)*

30g Parmesan cheese or cheddar, grated to serve

1. Preheat the oven to 180°C fan/ 200°C/400°F/ gas mark 6 and line a medium baking tray with baking paper.

2. Next, make the tomato sauce. Add 1 tablespoon of olive oil to a medium saucepan, add the onion and cook for 5–10 minutes until softened. Add the pepper and cook for 2 minutes. Add the tomatoes, swill a splash of water around the can and add this too,

together with two of the smashed garlic cloves, the oregano, chilli flakes and a pinch of salt.

3. Bring the sauce to the boil, then reduce the heat to low and keep at a gentle simmer for 25–30 minutes until the sauce has thickened. Stir occasionally and, after 15 minutes, use a wooden spoon to crush the tomatoes and garlic against the sides of the pan.

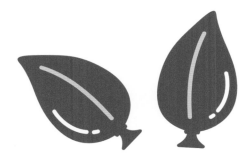

4. Next, add the sourdough to a blender and pulse to breadcrumbs. Transfer to a mixing bowl, then add the chickpeas, sun-dried tomatoes, basil leaves and remaining garlic clove to the blender and blitz to a paste. Add the paste to the sourdough crumbs in the mixing bowl, season generously and mix to combine. Create a well in the mixture, add the egg, use a fork to whisk and combine into the chickpea mixture. Separate the mixture into eight portions and roll into small balls.

5. Heat a medium frying pan over a medium heat and add the remaining tablespoon of olive oil. Tip in the chickpea balls and lightly brown on all sides for 3–5 minutes, before transferring to the lined baking tray and baking for 15 minutes.

6. Remove the tomato sauce from the heat and, using a stick blender, blend to a smooth sauce. Season to taste.

7. To serve, divide the chickpea balls between two plates and top with the tomato sauce, pesto and the Parmesan or cheddar, if using.

Leftover chickpea balls, sauce and pesto will keep in the fridge for up to 3 days.

mac 'n' cheese

Our Mum's go-to dish for us when we're home, here we've added some gut-loving twists to it. Lisa x

45 minutes | Serves 6

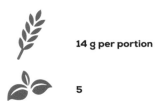

14 g per portion

5

allergens: *gluten, milk, nuts (cashews)*

60g (2¼ oz) cashews

2 tbsp olive oil

3 shallots, quartered

1 medium butternut squash *(skin on)*, cut into 2.5cm (1-in) cubes

1 parsnip *(skin on)*, roughly chopped

300g (10½ oz) dried pasta

300ml (10 fl oz) water

2–4 tbsp nutritional yeast

1 tbsp dried sage

60g (2¼ oz) feta cheese, crumbled (optional)

salt and pepper

Fibre – use wholegrain pasta
Variety – top with rocket
Ferments – try with a side of sauerkraut *(see page 256)*

1. To soak the cashews, place them in a bowl and cover with 2.5cm (1 in) of boiling water for 15 minutes, then drain.

2. Preheat the oven to 200°C fan/220°C/425°F/gas mark 7.

3. Put the butternut squash and parsnip on a baking tray, coat in the olive oil and season. Bake for 30–35 minutes until tender and golden. After 15 minutes, stir the vegetables and add the shallots for the final 15–20 minutes of cooking.

4. Cook the pasta according to the packet instructions, then drain and set aside.

5. Add the butternut squash, parsnip and shallots to a blender, along with the cashews and water, and blitz to a smooth sauce. Add the nutritional yeast and the sage and blend. Taste the sauce, add more nutritional yeast if needed and blend. Season to taste.

6. Pour the sauce over the cooked pasta and stir thoroughly to combine. Divide between bowls and sprinkle with the feta, if using. Serve immediately.

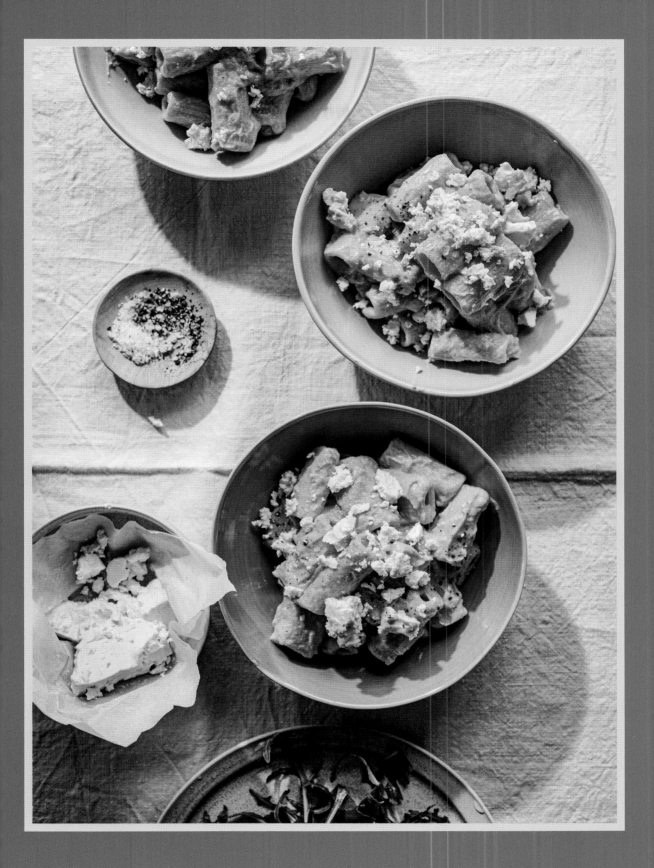

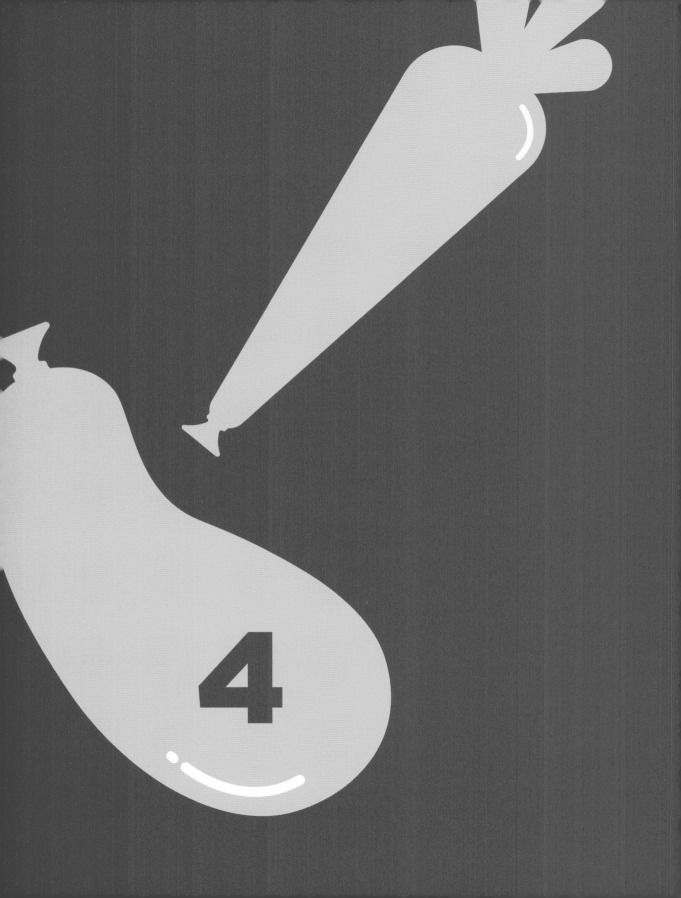

sides 'n' sauces

kefir tzatziki and sweet potato wedges

Break away from the usual suspects of BBQ sides – so so fresh and perfect for sharing. Lisa x

40 minutes | Serves 2

 1g per portion

 7

 milk kefir yogurt

allergens: *cow's milk*

KEFIR TZATZIKI

1 cucumber

1 small garlic clove, finely grated

squeeze of lemon juice

½ tsp paprika

½ x 400g (14-oz) can of chickpeas, drained and rinsed

handful of fresh flat-leaf parsley, roughly chopped

250g (9 oz) milk kefir yogurt *(homemade, see page 264, or shop-bought)*

SWEET POTATO WEDGES

2 sweet potatoes *(skin on)*, cut into wedges

1 tbsp olive oil

salt and pepper

1. Preheat the oven to 180°C fan/200°C/400°F/gas mark 6.

2. Scatter the sweet potatoes wedges over a baking tray, drizzle with olive oil, season and cook for 35–40 minutes until golden.

3. For the tzatziki, grate the cucumber and squeeze out the liquid, then mix with the garlic, lemon juice, paprika, chickpeas and most of the parsley and stir into the milk kefir yogurt until well combined. Season to taste and garnish with a little extra parsley and a drizzle of extra virgin olive oil. Serve with the sweet potato wedges.

Store in the fridge for up to 3 days.

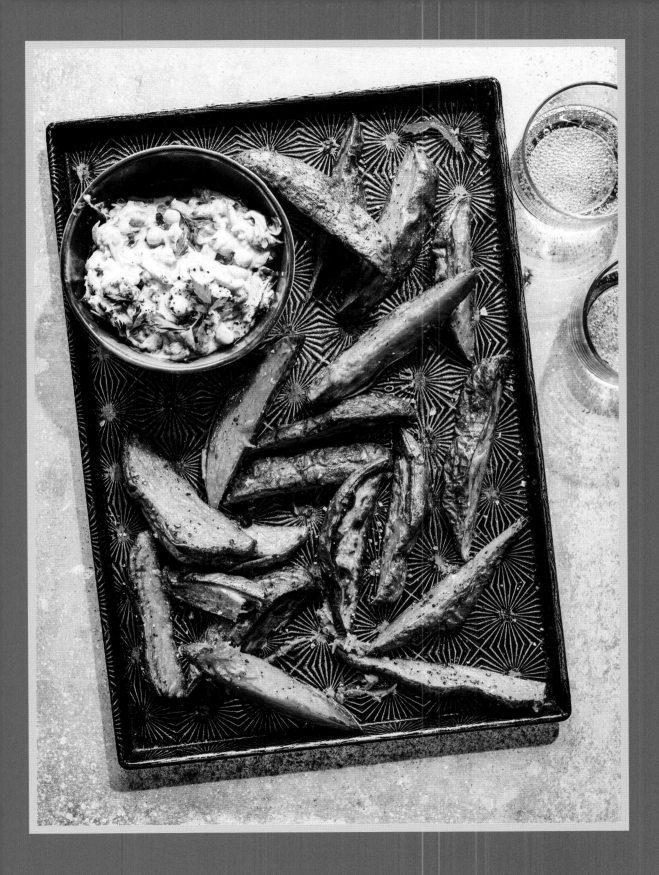

hummus

Hummus – lots of ways – sometimes I like to make them all at once for the ultimate dip fest... The chocolate suggestion came from one of our followers, Misty – love it with strawberries! Alana x

5 minutes | Serves 4

3.2g per portion

minimum 5

milk kefir yogurt

allergens: *cow's milk, sesame*

BASE HUMMUS

1 x 400g (14-oz) can of chickpeas, drained and rinsed

2–4 tbsp extra virgin olive oil

1 small garlic clove, smashed

½ tsp ground cumin

1 tbsp tahini

4 tbsp milk kefir yogurt
 (*homemade, see page 264 or shop-bought*)

zest and juice of ½ lemon

salt and pepper

....

1. Add the chickpeas and 2 tablespoons of the olive oil to a blender and blitz until smooth. Add the garlic, cumin, tahini, kefir and lemon juice and half the zest. Season before blending to a smooth paste, adding a little extra oil if required. Taste and add more lemon juice, zest and seasoning if required.

flavour combos

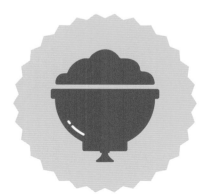

BEETS *Fibre – 3.5g per portion*

1 medium cooked beetroot

2a. Roughly slice the beetroot into wedges and add to the blender along with the chickpeas. Proceed as before.

....

BLACK BEAN AND LIME

Fibre – 5.7g per portion

½ x 400g (14-oz) can of black
    beans, drained and rinsed
½ tsp ground coriander *(to
    replace the cumin)*
zest and juice of ½ lime *(to
    replace the lemon)*
handful of fresh coriander,
    chopped

2b. Add the black beans to the blender with the chickpeas. Add the coriander and lime and proceed as in the main recipe. Top with the fresh coriander.

....

CHOCOLATE

Fibre – 4.4g per portion

1 tbsp cacao powder
2 tbsp honey or maple syrup

2c. Omit the garlic, cumin and lemon. Add the cacao and maple syrup with the tahini and kefir as for the base recipe.

GREEN *Fibre – 4g per portion*

handful of greens, such
    as spinach, rocket or
    watercress
50g jarred Jerusalem
    artichoke, drained

2d. Add the greens to the blender with the base ingredients and blend – an easy way to add variety!

....

TOMATO AND BASIL

Fibre – 4.9g per portion

50g (1¾ oz) sun-dried
    tomatoes
½ bunch of basil

2e. Add the sun-dried tomatoes and basil to the blender with the chickpeas and omit the cumin and tahini from the base recipe.

....

SMASHED WHITE BEAN

Fibre – 4.9g per portion

1 x 400g (14-oz) can of cannellini
    beans, drained and rinsed

2f. Add the cannellini beans to the blender with the chickpeas and proceed as for the main recipe.

Store in the fridge for up to 4 days.

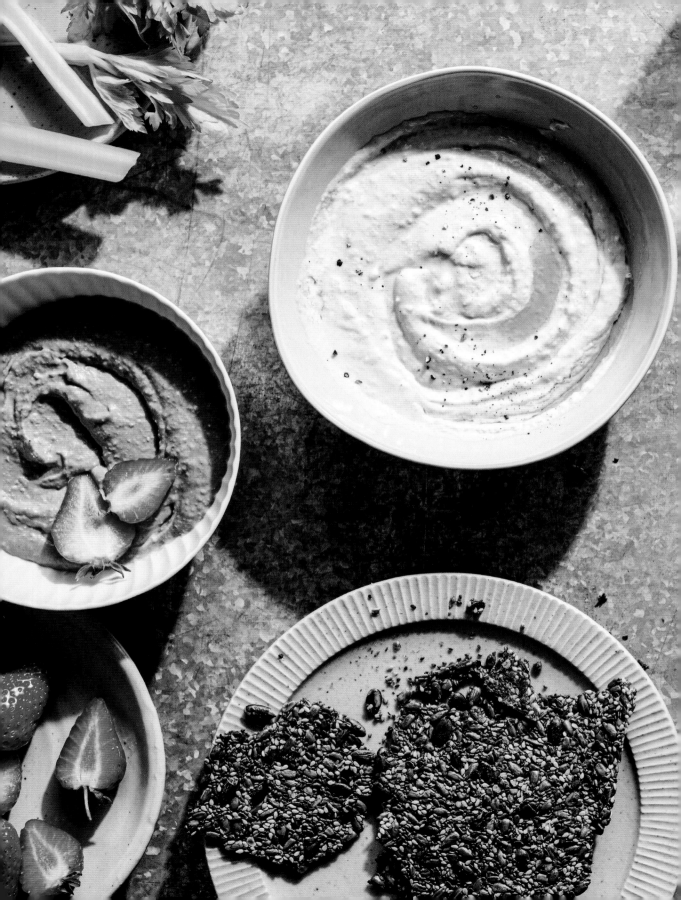

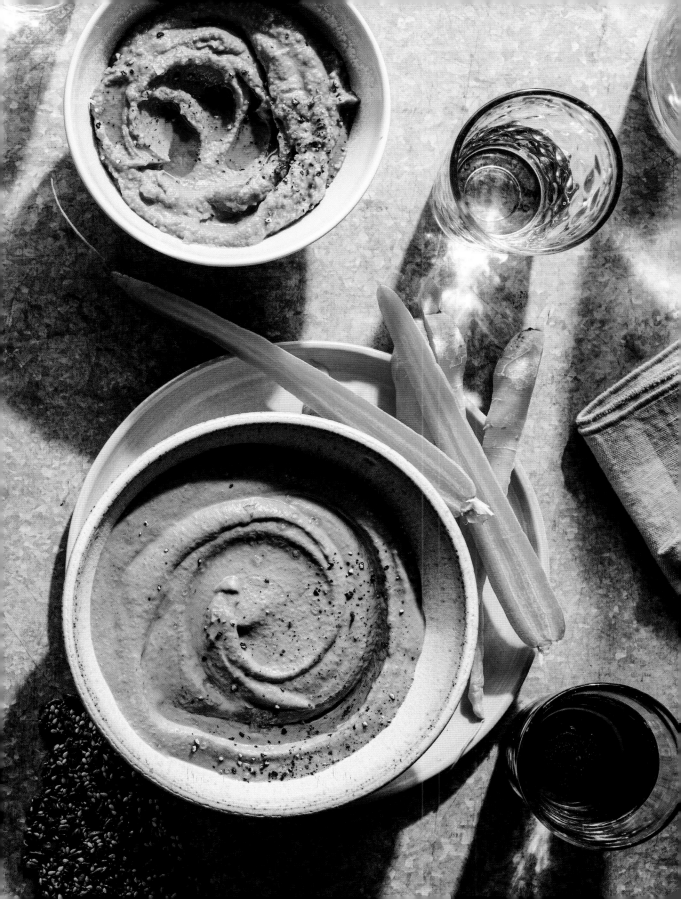

citrus greens

The best thing about dinners is all the sides and I always take it so far that there's never enough room on the table. However, the following dishes are designed to increase variety and fibre so you've got to make room for 'em all. Lisa x

15 minutes | Serves 4

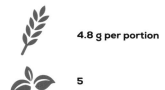

4.8 g per portion

5

allergens: *nuts (almonds)*

200g (7 oz) cavolo nero

1 tbsp olive oil

2 handfuls of broccoli (fresh or frozen), cut into florets

1 garlic clove, finely sliced or crushed

1 red or green chilli, deseeded and finely sliced

zest and juice of 1 orange

handful of flaked almonds

salt and pepper

1. Pull the green leaves of the cavolo nero away from the woody stalks and roughly shred, then discard the stalks.

2. Add the olive oil to a medium saucepan over a medium heat. Add the broccoli and a splash of water, then cover and cook for 3 minutes. Add the garlic and chilli and fry for a minute, afterwards adding the cavolo nero and season. Cover with a lid, cook for 2 minutes, stir, then cover again and cook for a further 2–4 minutes until the broccoli is tender and the cavolo nero is wilted.

3. Add the orange zest, a squeeze of orange juice and top with the flaked almonds. Serve immediately.

sliced root vegetable bake

Follows the simplicity of a traditional roast and, as with all roasts, it's all in the timings baby! Alana x

1 hour | Serves 4–6 as a side

minimum 5.4g
per portion

5

allergens: *gluten (check shop-bought vegetable stock)*

2 tbsp olive oil

1 kg (2 lb 4 oz) mix of root vegetables, such as potatoes, sweet potatoes, turnips, beetroot or parsnips, cut into 5mm (¼ in) thick rounds *(using a mandolin will make slicing easier)*

5 garlic cloves, smashed

500ml (18 fl oz) vegetable stock or water

2 tbsp fresh or dried mixed herbs, such as rosemary, thyme or sage

salt and pepper

1. Preheat the oven to 180°C fan/200°C/400°F/gas mark 6.

2. Grease a medium baking dish with a little of the olive oil. Layer the root veg into the dish, alternating between the different types. Once they are tightly packed, add the stock or water to fill the dish halfway and slot the smashed garlic cloves in between the vegetables. Season well.

3. Brush the top of the vegetables with the remaining oil and sprinkle over the mixed herbs. Cover with foil and bake for 30–35 minutes. Once the vegetables have started to soften, remove the foil and cook for a further 20 minutes until golden.

potato salad with sauerkraut

This is your new BBQ go-to – the perfect cut-through for those sweet and smokey BBQ flavours. Lisa x

30 minutes | 2 as a main or 4 as a side

11g per mains portion

10 *(based on 3 different types in the mixed-leaf bag)*

sauerkraut

small bunch of fresh basil, leaves picked

500g (1lb 2 oz) new potatoes

120g (4¼ oz) frozen peas

3–4 tbsp extra virgin olive oil

1 small garlic clove

2 handfuls of mixed leaf salad

2 spring onions, finely sliced

bunch of fresh flat-leaf parsley, chopped

6 radishes, sliced

120g (4¼ oz) sauerkraut *(homemade, see page 256, or shop-bought)*

salt and pepper

1. Bring a large pan of salted water to the boil, drop in the basil and blanch for 20 seconds, then remove with a slotted spoon and set aside to cool.

2. Slice any large potatoes in half and add along with the rest to the pan of boiling salted water and cook for 20 minutes until tender, adding the peas for the final 3 minutes. Drain and leave to steam-dry while you make the basil dressing.

3. Squeeze any liquid from the basil, then add the leaves to a blender along with the oil and garlic. Blitz until you have a vibrant green oil.

4. Put the potatoes, peas, mixed leaf salad, spring onions and parsley in a mixing bowl and toss with the basil oil. Add the sliced radishes and season to taste. Serve topped with sauerkraut.

Store any leftovers in the fridge for up to 3 days.

butternut squash and lentil stuffing

This filling is not just for Christmas... Alana x

1 hour+ | Serves 4–6 as a side

 7.9g per portion

 6

 sauerkraut

allergens: *gluten, nuts (walnuts)*

2 tbsp butter or olive oil, plus extra for greasing

2 slices of day-old sourdough (*homemade, see page 252, or shop-bought*)

1 red onion, finely diced

1 tbsp dried sage

1 medium butternut squash, (*skin on*) cut into 2.5cm (1-in) cubes, seeds reserved

2–3 garlic cloves, crushed

1 x 250g packet cooked Puy lentils

400ml (14 fl oz) vegetable or chicken stock

2 sprigs of fresh thyme

4 tbsp dried cranberries (*optional*)

handful of walnuts, roughly chopped

salt and pepper

1. Preheat the oven to 180°C fan/ 200°C/400°F/gas mark 6 and grease a medium baking dish with butter or oil.

2. Lightly toast the sourdough before tearing it into small pieces. Set aside.

3. Add 1 tablespoon of the butter or olive oil to a large non-stick pan over a medium-high heat. Add the onion and soften for 5 minutes, then add the butternut squash. Season well and add the dried sage. Cook for 10 minutes until the squash begins to soften. Stir in the remaining butter or oil, add the garlic and cook for a further 2 minutes. Remove from the heat and transfer to a medium bowl. Add the toasted sourdough and lentils, then add the stock.

4. Transfer the mixture to the greased baking dish, add the thyme and cover with foil. Cook in the oven for 30 minutes, then remove the foil and scatter over the butternut squash seeds, walnuts and cranberries (if using) and cook for a further 15–20 minutes until golden and crispy.

mushy peas

You mustn't have your TGS fish and chips without it… Lisa x

15 minutes | Serves 4

9g per portion

4

milk kefir yogurt

allergens: cow's milk

1 tbsp butter

1 x 400g (14-oz) can of cannellini beans, drained and rinsed

400g (14 oz) frozen peas

squeeze of lemon juice

2 tbsp milk kefir yogurt (home-made, see page 264, or shop-bought)

handful of fresh mint leaves, roughly chopped

salt and pepper

1. Add the butter to medium saucepan over a medium-high heat, add the cannellini beans and season well. Reduce the heat and add the peas. Cook for 5 minutes until cooked through. Add the lemon juice.

2. Mash the beans and peas by hand until they have reached your desired consistency. Stir through the kefir yogurt and mint and season to taste before serving.

tartare sauce

Tartare sauce… but not as you know it… Lisa x

10 minutes | Serves 4

1g per portion

5

milk kefir yogurt and olives

allergens: milk

1 small shallot, finely diced

6 tbsp milk kefir yogurt (home-made, see page 264, or shop-bought)

1 tsp capers, finely chopped

handful of stoned olives, finely chopped

handful of fresh parsley

squeeze of lemon juice

salt and pepper

1. Add the shallot, milk kefir yogurt, capers, olives and parsley to a bowl and mix to combine. Add a squeeze of lemon and season to taste.

Store in the fridge for up to 2 days.

slaw

I have coleslaw with EVERYTHING (it was always such a luxury when we were younger) and after this, you will too. Lisa x

15 minutes | Serves 4

4.1g per portion

minimum 3

milk kefir yogurt

allergens: *cow's milk*

....

2 carrots (*skin on*)
½ cabbage (*white, green or red or a mix*)
handful of fresh flat-leaf parsley

2–4 tbsp milk kefir yogurt (*homemade, see page 264, or shop-bought*)
1 tbsp apple cider vinegar
salt and pepper

....

1. Grate the carrots, shred the cabbage and roughly chop the parsley.

2. Add all the ingredients to a bowl, mix well and season to taste.

Store in the fridge for up to 3 days.

corn salsa

Who knew sweetcorn could add such pizzazz to salsa? A great add-on to our spiced bean and jackfruit tacos (see page 194). Alana x

5 minutes | Serves 4

2g per portion

5

....

2 handfuls of cherry tomatoes, halved
4 spring onions, sliced
1 x 160g (5½-oz) can of sweetcorn, drained

1 red chilli, deseeded and finely chopped
squeeze of fresh lime juice
salt and pepper

....

1. Put all the ingredients in a mixing bowl, add a squeeze of lime juice, stir well and season to taste.

Store leftovers in the fridge for up to 3 days.

fermented tomato ketchup

For all the ketchup fiends in your house – your gut bugs will be hooked on it too. Makes perfect condi-sense. Lisa x

15 minutes prep | Serves 30+

and up to 5 days fermentation

 minimum 6

allergens: *mustard*

500g (1 lb 2 oz) passata

150g (5½ oz) jarred tomato purée

2 garlic cloves

2 tbsp kombucha *(with mother, homemade, see page 266, or shop-bought)* or brine from existing vegetable ferments

1 tsp onion powder

1 tsp allspice

½ tsp mustard powder

50ml (2 fl oz) apple cider vinegar

50ml (2 fl oz) maple syrup

½ tsp salt

pepper, to taste

1. Add all the ingredients to a large mixing bowl and stir to combine. Transfer to a 1-litre (1¾-pint) jar and seal with a burping lid. Leave at room temperature out of direct sunlight for five days. Begin taste testing from day three and, once the tomato ketchup has reached your desired flavour, replace the burping lid with a screw-top lid.

Store in the fridge for up to 3 months.

fermented hot sauce

Get this right on some cheese on toast... or anything really. In fact, keep a bottle in your handbag. Lisa x

10 minutes prep | makes 1 litre

+ 7–14 days fermentation

 3

800ml (1½ pints) water

3 tbsp sea salt

500g (1 lb 2 oz) red chillies, stalks removed and halved

2 Scotch bonnet chillies, stalks removed and halved *(optional)*

6 garlic cloves, peeled

50g (1¾ oz) fresh or frozen fruit, defrosted, such as blueberries, strawberries or mixed berries

1. Wash a 1 litre (1¾ pints) jar in hot soapy water, then place it in the oven at 90°C fan/110°C/225°F/gas mark ¼ for 15–20 minutes to sterilize it. Leave it to cool.

2. Place the water and salt in a jug and stir to dissolve to create a brine. Add the chillies, garlic and fruit to the sterilized jar and pour in the brine, ensuring the chillies are submerged.

3. Cover the jar with a burping lid and leave it to sit at room temperature, out of direct sunlight, for 7–14 days until you can smell a pleasant sour smell.

4. Strain the brine and reserve it. Transfer the chillies, garlic and fruit to a blender with 100ml (3½ fl oz) brine. Blitz until you have a smooth sauce consistency, using the remaining brine to loosen if required. Return the hot sauce to a clean 1 litre (1¾ pints) jar and cover with a screw-top lid.

Store in the fridge for up to 3 months.

piccalilli

I was actually surprised at how many different types of veg are in Piccalilli, your variety sandwich GO TO. Lisa x

10 minutes prep | makes 1 litre
+ 4 hours resting
+ 5–14 days fermentation

 10

allergens: *mustard*

- **1** small cauliflower, cut into florets
- **1** medium courgette, halved and sliced
- **2 handfuls** of green beans, trimmed and halved
- **1** red pepper, cored, deseeded and sliced
- **80ml (2¾ fl oz)** water
- **2 tbsp** honey or maple syrup
- **20g (¾ oz)** rice flour
- **1 tbsp** mustard powder
- **1 tbsp** mustard seeds
- **2 tsp** ground cumin
- **1 tsp** coriander seeds
- **1 tsp** ground turmeric
- sea salt

1. Wash a 1-litre jar in hot soapy water, then place it in the oven at 90°C fan/110°C/225°F/gas mark ¼ for 15–20 minutes to sterilize it. Leave it to cool.

2. Place a mixing bowl on a set of scales and zero the scales. Place the vegetables in the bowl and measure their weight. Calculate 2% of that weight (by multiplying by 0.02) and measure out the result in salt. Sprinkle the measured salt over the vegetables and gently mix. This will begin to draw water out of the vegetables. Leave to sit for 4 hours.

3. To make the sauce, add the water, honey and rice flour to a saucepan over a medium heat. Bring to the boil and leave to thicken. Remove from the heat and leave to cool.

4. Mix the spices together and add with the sauce to the vegetables, gently massaging through (it's a good idea to wear gloves here so the turmeric doesn't stain your hands!). Pack the vegetables into the sterilized jar, pressing down so that the spice sauce covers the vegetables.

5. Cover the jar with a burping lid and leave it at room temperature, out of direct sunlight. After 24 hours, press down the vegetables again. Begin to taste test after five days. Once the piccalilli has reached your desired tanginess, replace the burping lid with a screw-top lid, and securely cover.

Store in the fridge for up to 3 months.

crunchy seed and nut mix

Make em and shake em.. the easiest way to add variety to any dish. Alana x

25 minutes | Serves 10

2.7g per tbsp

minimum 7

allergens: *nuts (hazelnuts, walnuts, almonds, cashews or pistachios), sesame*

120g (3½ oz) mixed nuts, such as hazelnuts, walnuts, almonds, cashews or pistachios

100g (1¾ oz) mixed seeds, such as pumpkin, sunflower and flaxseed

2 tbsp sesame seeds

1 tbsp cumin seeds

1 tbsp coriander seeds

1 tbsp fennel seeds

pinch of chilli flakes *(optional)*

salt and pepper

1. Preheat the oven to 180°C fan/200°C/400°F/gas mark 6.

2. Spread the nuts and mixed seeds (except the sesame seeds) over a baking tray and cook for 10–15 minutes until toasted.

3. Put a small non-stick pan over a medium heat. Add the sesame, cumin, coriander and fennel seeds and toast for 2 minutes. Remove from the heat, roughly chop the nuts and grind the toasted spices with a pestle and mortar. Mix the spices into the nuts.

4. Sprinkle over hot dishes, traybakes, hummus, dips or salads.

Store at room temperature in an airtight container for up to 2 weeks.

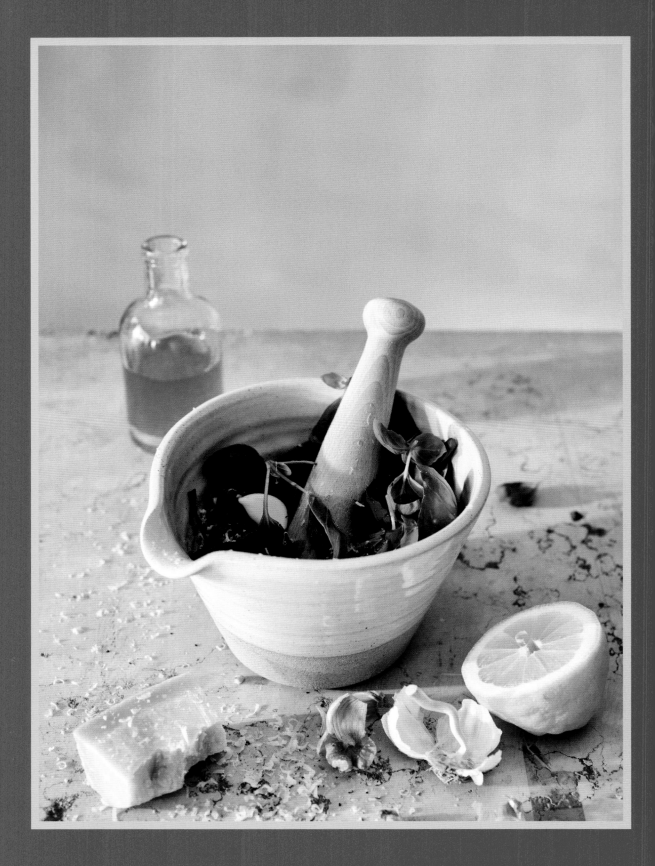

walnut pesto

I always get a big jar and make a double batch to add to meals for a variety-filled taste sensation. Lisa x

10 minutes | Serves 2

2.1g per portion

5

allergens: *nuts (walnuts), cow's milk (if using Parmesan)*

60g (2¼ oz) walnuts

1 small garlic clove, peeled

small bunch of fresh basil, leaves only

zest and juice of ½ lemon

2–4 tbsp extra virgin olive oil

2 handfuls of rocket or spinach

2 tbsp grated Parmesan cheese or 3 tbsp nutritional yeast

salt and pepper

1. Add the walnuts to a small pan over a medium-high heat and toast for a couple of minutes on each side. Remove from the heat, leave to cool for 2 minutes and then add to a blender. Blitz until coarsely chopped, about 10 seconds, then add the garlic, basil leaves, lemon zest, salt and pepper and gradually add the extra virgin olive oil to bind. Season to taste.

Store in the fridge for up to 4 days or in the freezer for up to a month.

just
desserts

summer trifle

Trifle made with butterbeans – YEAH YOU HEARD IT. Alana x

30 minutes | Serves 4–6
+ cooling

 8.2g per portion

 minimum 6

 milk kefir yogurt

allergens: *cow's milk, nuts (almonds and pitachios), eggs*

CAKE LAYER

1 x 400g (14-oz) can of butterbeans, drained and rinsed

2 tbsp maple syrup

2 eggs, beaten

50g ground almonds

1 tsp baking powder

½ tsp salt

25g coconut oil, melted

FRUIT JAM LAYER

300g (7 oz) fresh, frozen mango or frozen tropical fruit mix

2 tbsp chia seeds

TO SERVE

2 kiwis, sliced

8 tbsp milk kefir yogurt *homemade, see page 264, or shop-bought)*

2 tbsp pistachios, roughly chopped

---

1. To make the cake layer, preheat the oven to 180°C fan/200°C/400°F/gas mark 6. Line a 20cm (8-in) cake tin with baking paper.

2. Put the butterbeans and maple syrup into a food processor and purée until smooth, whilst gradually adding the eggs.

3. Transfer the puréed mixture to a mixing bowl and fold in the ground almonds, baking powder, salt and coconut oil. Once combined tip into the lined cake tin and place to the oven for 20 minutes until golden on top. Set aside to cool.

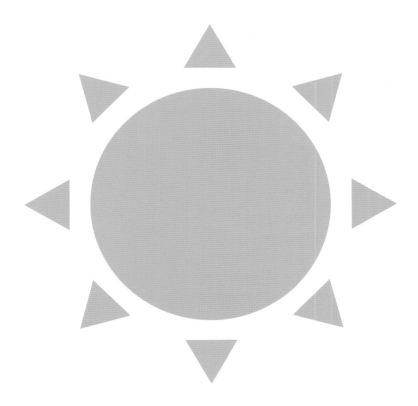

4. Meanwhile, make the fruit chia jam. Place the fruit in a small saucepan with 100ml (3½ fl oz) water over a low heat, stirring occasionally, until the fruit begins to break down. Use a masher to mash the fruit to your desired consistency (or a food processor to pulse the fruit if you prefer a smoother consistency). Stir in the chia seeds until combined. Remove from the heat and leave to cool to room temperature.

5. Once the cake has cooled, crumble half between 4–6 pots, then layer with half the fruit jam and a spoonful of milk kefir yogurt. Repeat with another layer of cake, fruit jam and kefir and then top with the sliced kiwis and chopped pistachios.

Store in the fridge for up to a day. The fruit chia jam can be stored for up to 5 days if stored separately in an airtight container.

banoffee pie with kefir

MY FAVOURITE DESSERT! The last time I made this, my dog ate the base as it was cooling in the garden, so keep it indoors ha! Lisa x

40 minutes | Serves 6

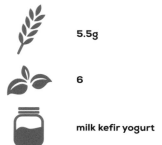

5.5g

6

milk kefir yogurt

allergens: *nuts (almonds), cow's milk, gluten*

OATY BASE

80g rolled oats

2 tbsp coconut oil

1 ripe banana

1 tsp ground cinnamon

½ tbsp cacao powder

pinch of sea salt

2 tbsp smooth peanut butter

DATE FILLING

200g (7 oz) stoned Medjool or soft dates

TOPPING

4 tbsp milk kefir yogurt *(homemade, see page 264, or shop-bought)*

1 large ripe banana, sliced into rounds

20g (¾ oz) 70% cocoa solids dark chocolate, cut into shavings

---

1. Preheat the oven to 180°C fan/200°C/400°F/gas mark 6. Place the dates in a bowl and cover in warm water. Leave to soak for 15 minutes, then drain, add to a blender and blitz to a paste.

2. While the dates are soaking, place the oats in a food processor and pulse until roughly ground. Place the coconut oil in a small saucepan and melt over a low heat.

3. Place the oats, cinnamon, cacao and salt in a mixing bowl and stir to combine. Add the banana and mash with a fork, then add the coconut oil and peanut butter and stir to combine.

4. Once mixed, line a 20cm (8-in) cake tin with baking paper (if using a cake tin with a removable base, there's no need to line it). Add the cake mix and bake for 15–20 minutes until golden. Remove from the oven and leave to cool.

5. To build the pie, spread the date paste over the oaty base, top with the sliced bananas, drizzle with milk kefir yogurt and finish with a sprinkle of dark chocolate shavings. Cool in the fridge before removing from the tin and cut into slices before serving.

The banana will begin to brown quite quickly, so store in the fridge and eat within a day.

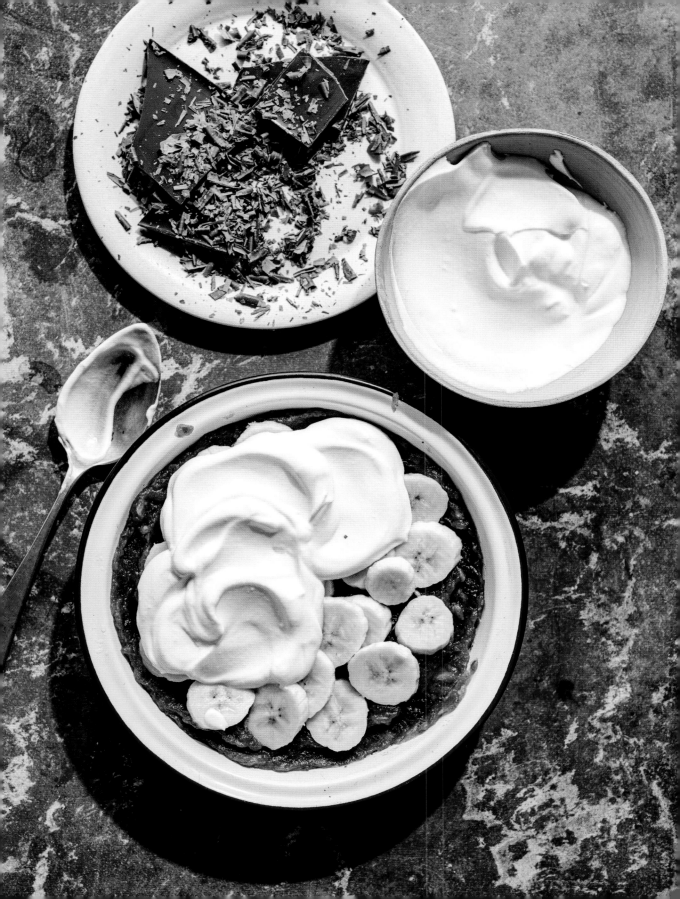

fruit crumble

The perfect end to a Sunday roast! Alana x

40 minutes | Serves 4–6

5.1g per portion

6

milk kefir yogurt

allergens: *gluten, cow's milk*

4 apples *(skin on)*, roughly chopped

1 pear *(skin on)*, roughly chopped

100ml (3½ fl oz) water

100g (3½ oz) rolled oats

1 tsp ground cinnamon

1 tbsp maple syrup

1 tbsp coconut oil, melted

milk kefir yogurt *(homemade see page 264, or shop-bought)* or dairy-free alternative, to serve

1. Preheat the oven to 180°C fan/200°C/400°F/gas mark 6.

2. Place the apple, pears and water in a deep, heavy-based pan over a low-medium heat. Cook gently for 15 minutes until softened.

3. Add the oats, cinnamon, maple syrup and coconut oil to a mixing bowl and stir to combine.

4. Spread the fruit mixture over the base of a baking dish. Top with the oat mix and bake for 15–20 minutes until the oats are golden. To serve, top the crumble with a spoonful of milk kefir yogurt.

Leftover crumble can be stored in the fridge for up to 3 days and reheated before serving.

 Fibre and Variety – *add a handful of frozen cranberries when you're cooking the apples and pears*

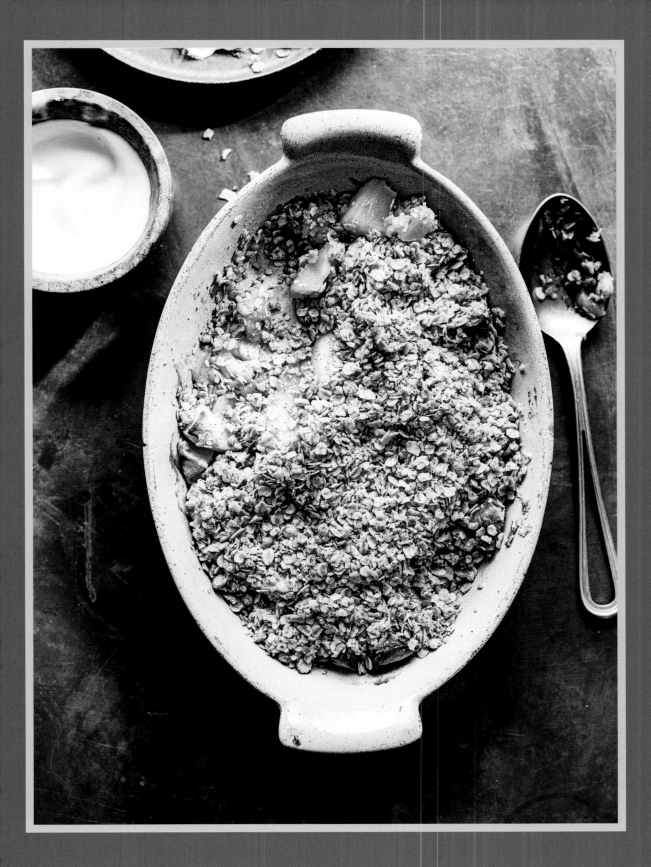

sauerkraut brownies

We know this is RANDOM, but don't knock 'em til you try 'em. Lisa x

10 minutes | Serves 8–10
+ 30 minutes cooling

 6.2g

 minimum 6

 sauerkraut

allergens: *nuts (almonds)*

60g (2¼ oz) sauerkraut *(homemade, see page 256, or shop-bought), finely chopped*

400g (14 oz) stoned Medjool or soft dates

80g (2¾ oz) ground almonds

3 tbsp cacao powder

½ tsp sea salt

handful of walnuts, roughly chopped

80g (2¾ oz) mixed seeds *(pumpkin, sunflower, sesame, flaxseed or linseed)*

1. Using a chopping board, finely chop the sauerkraut. Use kitchen paper to remove any excess liquid.

2. Place the dates, ground almonds, mixed seeds, cacao and salt in a food processor and blend until the mixture starts to stick together. Mix in the sauerkraut.

3. Line a square brownie tin with baking paper. Tip in the brownie mix and press firmly into the dish with your hands until evenly distributed.

4. Once the mix is evenly distributed, press the walnuts into the top of the brownies. Transfer to the fridge to set for 20–30 minutes. Remove the brownies from the fridge and cut into 8–10 squares.

Store in an airtight container in the fridge for up to 3 days.

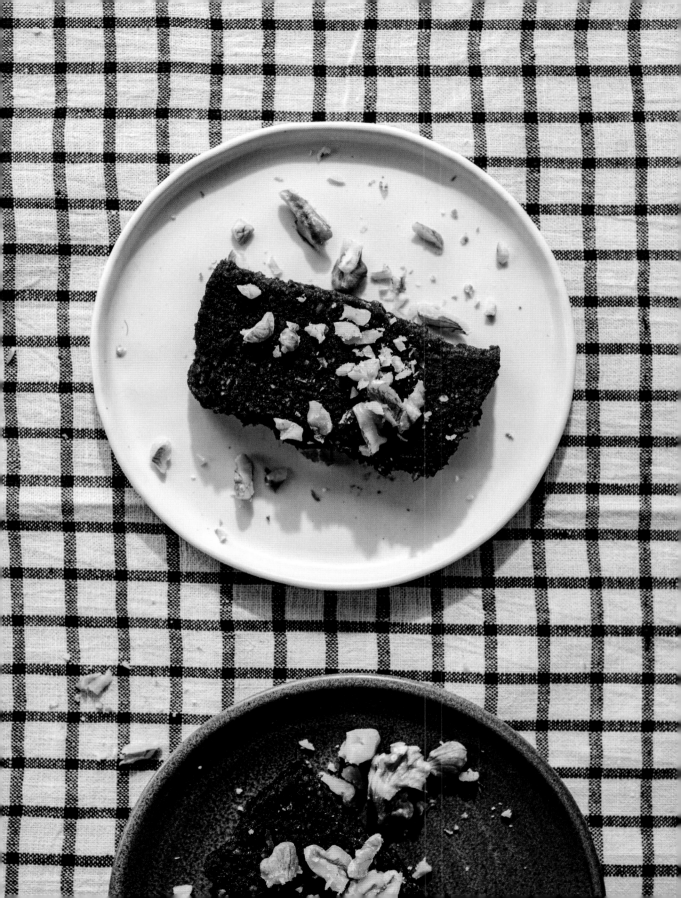

banana and raspberry cookies

An absolute WINNER with a cup of tea! Alana x

35 minutes | Makes 6

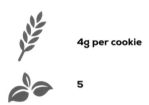

4g per cookie

5

allergens: *nuts (peanut, almond or cashew), gluten, cow's milk – milk kefir yogurt, if using*

2 medium, ripe bananas

135g (4¾ oz) rolled oats

1 tsp ground cinnamon

2 tbsp nut butter, such as peanut, almond or cashew

pinch of sea salt

2 handfuls of raspberries (fresh or frozen)

1. Preheat the oven to 170°C fan/190°C/ 375°F/gas mark 5 and line a baking tray with baking paper.

2. In a large bowl, use the back of a fork to mash the bananas, then add the oats, cinnamon, nut butter and salt and mix to combine. Finally add the raspberries and gently combine. Use your hands to roll the mixture into 6–8 balls, then transfer to the lined baking tray and press down into cookies.

3. Bake for 20–25 minutes until golden. Eat warm or leave to cool on a wire rack.

Once cool, store in the fridge for up to 4 days.

Fibre – *add a handful of chopped walnuts*
Variety – *top with mixed seeds (pumpkin, sunflower, sesame, flaxseed or linseed)*
Ferment – *milk kefir yogurt (see page 264)*

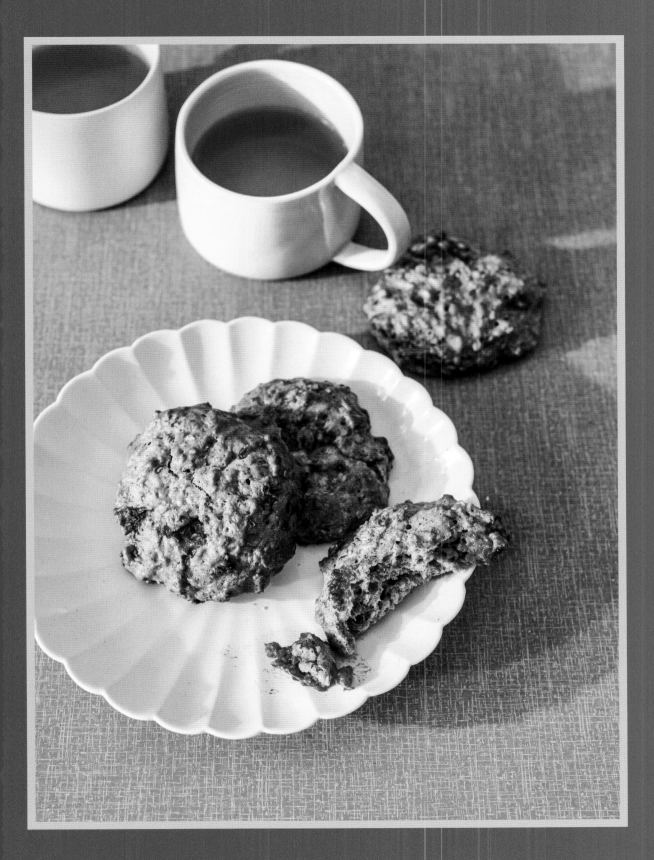

'nICE' cream and toppings

Ice cream, you scream, everybody scream (nicely!). Alana x

5 minutes | Serves 2

4.8g per portion

2

milk kefir

allergens: *cow's milk – milk kefir, if using*

2 frozen ripe bananas

1 frozen ripe avocado

250ml (9 fl oz) milk *(dairy, nut or plant-based or milk kefir)*

2 tbsp maple syrup

1 vanilla pod, deseeded (optional)

2 handfuls of ice cubes

TOPPINGS

80g raspberries
   (+5.4g fibre)

80g blueberries
   (+1.2g fibre)

80g strawberries
   (+3g fibre)

2 tbsp pumpkin seeds
   (+1.5g fibre)

2 tbsp sunflower seeds
   (+1.4g fibre)

2 tbsp chia seeds
   (+7.7g fibre)

2 tbsp chopped cashews
   (+1.6g fibre)

2 tbsp chopped almonds
   (+3.2g fibre)

1. Add all the ingredients to a blender and blend until smooth. This forms an instant 'nice' cream texture.

Either eat immediately or store in the freezer for up to a week.

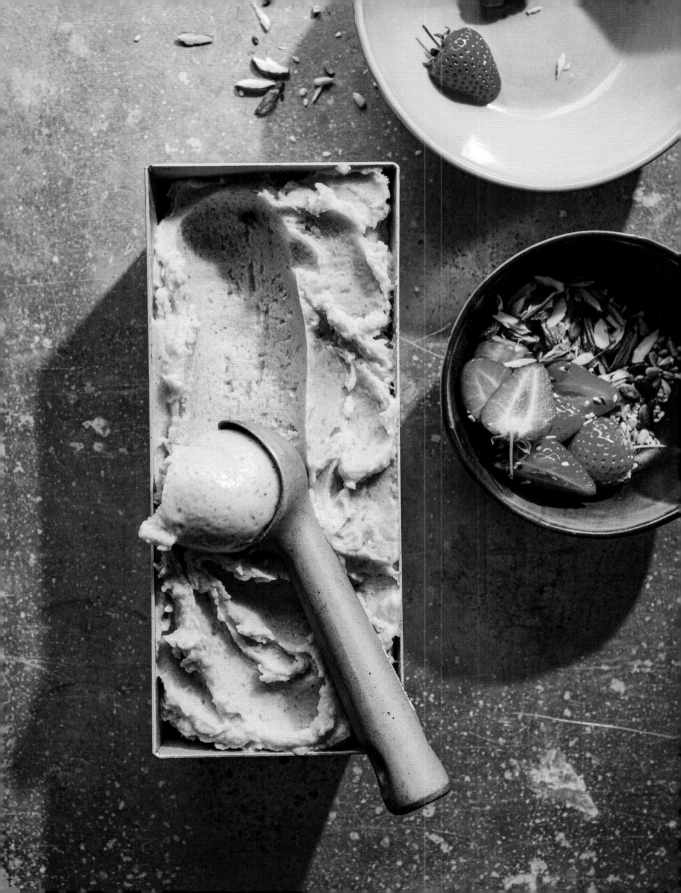

mocktails

Upgrade your soft drink with your gut in mind – take us to The Gut Stuff bar!!

Up to 3 days | Serves 4
after following first step fermentation (see kombucha page 266)

 2

 kombucha

beetroot and ginger kombucha

1 beetroot, peeled and chopped into 1cm (½-in) cubes (or 120ml/3¾ fl oz pressed beetroot juice)

800ml (1½ pints) kombucha from first fermentation *(see page 266)*

2 tbsp freshly grated, peeled ginger

. . . .

1. Preheat the oven to 180°C fan/200°C/400°F/gas mark 6.

2. If using beetroot, place it in the centre of a piece of foil, drizzle with 1 tablespoon of water and bring the sides of the foil together to create a parcel. Cook for 40 minutes.

3. Once the beetroot has cooled, transfer to a blender and purée into a smooth paste, adding a splash of kombucha.

4. Add the beetroot paste/juice and grated ginger to a 1 litre (1¾-pint) clip-top bottle. Using a funnel, pour in the first fermentation kombucha, leaving 2.5–5cm (1–2 in) clear at the top.

5. Store at room temperature, out of direct sunlight, for up to 3 days, until it reaches the desired level of carbonation. Chill in the fridge before serving.

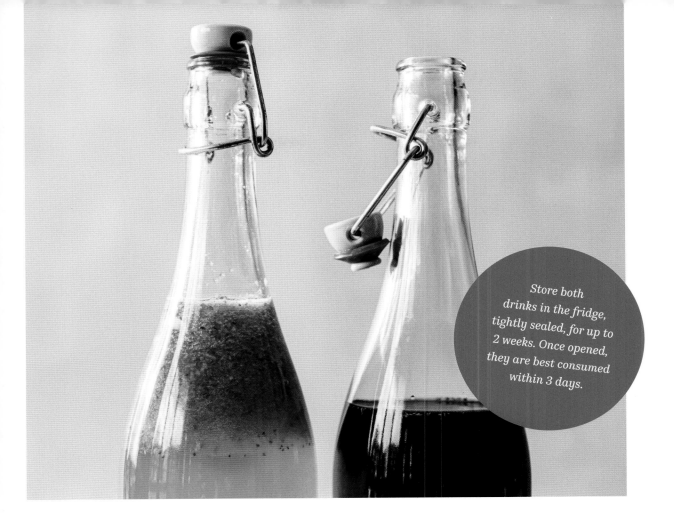

Store both drinks in the fridge, tightly sealed, for up to 2 weeks. Once opened, they are best consumed within 3 days.

Up to 2 days | serves 4

after following first step fermentation (See water kefir page 265)

2

water kefir

strawberry and lemongrass

50g (1¾ oz) strawberries, crushed

1 lemongrass stick, finely sliced

800ml (1½ pints) water kefir from first fermentation *(see page 265)*

. . . .

1. Add the strawberries and lemongrass to a 1 litre (1 ¾-pint) clip-top bottle. Using a funnel, pour in the water kefir, leaving 2.5–5cm (1–2 in) clear at the top.

2. Store at room temperature, out of direct sunlight, for up to 2 days until it reaches desired level of carbonation. Chill in the fridge before serving.

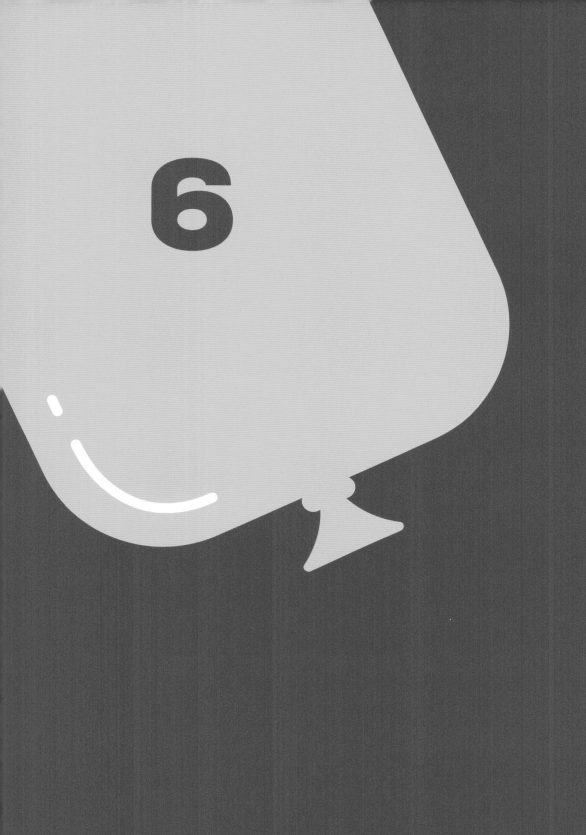

ferments

sourdough starter

7 days | Serves n/a
+ weekly feeds

allergens: *gluten*

500g (1 lb 2 oz) wholemeal
flour
500g (1 lb 2 oz) strong white
bread flour
1030ml (2 lb 5oz) water

We've set up all our ferments with dating profiles so you can choose which one you want to take to dinner first ;)

Weigh an empty 500ml (18-fl oz) jar and make a note of the weight.

Day 1 – To make the starter mixture, combine 50g (1¾ oz) wholemeal flour, 50g (1¾ oz) strong white flour and 125g (4½ oz) water (at 24°C/75°F) in a bowl. Transfer to the 500ml jar and cover with a two-part lid. Leave at room temperature for 24 hours.

Day 2 – Add 75g (2¾ oz) starter mixture to a bowl (discard the rest), followed by 50 g (1¾ oz) wholemeal flour, 50g (1¾ oz) strong white flour and 115g (4 oz) water (at 24°C/75°F). Mix well, return to the jar, cover and leave at room temperature for 24 hours.

Days 3 and 4 – Repeat day 2.

Day 5 – Increase the feed to twice a day. In the jar, reduce the starter (discard the rest) to 75g (2¾ oz), then add 50g (1¾ oz) wholemeal flour, 50g (1¾ oz) strong white flour and 115g (4 oz) water

(at 24°C/75°F). Mix well, cover and leave at room temperature for 12 hours. After 12 hours, repeat the feed with the same ratio of ingredients and set aside for 12 hours.

Day 6 – Repeat day 5.

Day 7 – Reduce the starter to 50g (1¾ oz), add 50g (1¾ oz) wholemeal flour, 50g (1¾ oz) strong white flour and 100g (3½ oz) water (at 24°C/75°F). After 12 hours, repeat the feed with the same ratio of ingredients and set aside for 12 hours.

After Day 7 – If you are not baking on a regular basis, store your starter in the fridge until you are ready to, and follow our weekly feeding instructions:

We recommend feeding the starter once a week whilst refrigerated. Feed it by first discarding all but 50g (1¾ oz) of the starter, then add 50g (1¾ oz) of wholemeal flour, 50g (1¾ oz) of strong white flour and 100g (3½ oz) water. Stir the mixture together with a spoon before replacing it to the fridge.

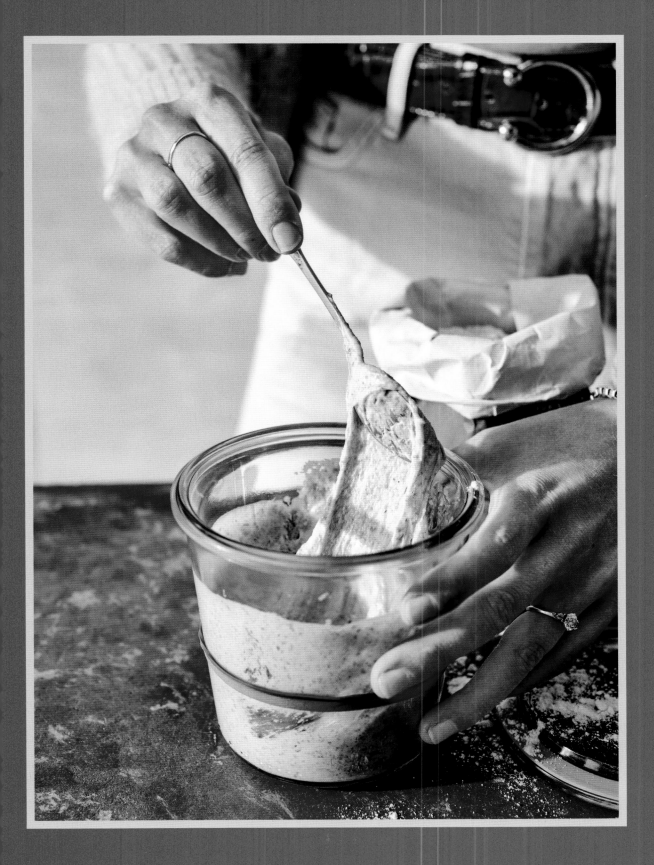

the gut stuff sourdough

Name: Sourdough (say it right 'sour-doh').

What is it: Bread made using a live starter instead of yeast to help it rise.

Flavour: Sour and tangy.

Likes: Flour, salt and water.

Dislikes: Not being fed enough flour (flangry – flour hangry).

Describe yourself in a few words: I'm moreish, have a good ear and you can put anything on top of me and I'll taste good.

Sophie Stensrud
We knew we HAD to ask Sophie to contribute to this book as she has cooked and baked all her life and runs baking classes via The Scandicook – there's nothin' she doesn't know about sourdough!

up to 36 hours | Serves 12–14 slices
including resting

allergens: *gluten*

100g (3½ oz) active starter
350g (12 oz) water
300g (10½ oz) strong white bread flour
150g (5½ oz) strong wholemeal flour
50g (1¾ oz) rye flour
10g (¼ oz) salt

Step 1 – Your starter needs to be active, stringy and bubbly and to have at least doubled when you start mixing the dough. Add the water and starter to a mixing bowl and mix well to dissolve the starter. Add the flour and mix until it is fully hydrated, and no dry bits remain. Cover the bowl and leave for 30 minutes–1 hour.

Step 2 – Sprinkle the salt over the dough, splash on a little water (about 1 tablespoon), and squish the salt into the dough with wet hands. You can then knead the dough on the counter for a few minutes using the 'slap and fold' method or mix really well in the bowl and then do a series of stretch and folds. To stretch and fold grab the dough at the top end of the bowl, pull it up then over towards the bottom of the bowl. Use the other hand to turn the bowl and repeat all the way round the bowl a few times until you feel the dough is uniform and starting to tighten up a little. Cover the bowl again and leave it to rest for about 30 minutes.

Step 3 – Roughly every 30 minutes (or when the dough has relaxed back into the bowl) do a set of stretch and folds around the bowl, 4–6 stretches. Repeat 3–6 times.

Step 4 – Leave your covered bowl to rest and finish bulk proving. How long this takes depends on temperature and how active your starter is, it could be anything from 3–8 hours in total from adding the salt. When finished your dough should have increased in size about 50% – it should dome a little, be glossy and have some visible air bubbles.

Step 5 – Pre-shape by tipping the dough onto the countertop and, using a damp dough scraper and damp hands, shape it into a round. Leave to bench rest for about 30 minutes.

Step 6 – Prep your banneton, or a bowl covered with a tea towel by dusting it well with rice flour to avoid the dough sticking.

Lightly flour the dough and the counter next to it, as well as your hands. Using a dough scraper, flip your round upside down onto the flour.

Shaping a batard (oval loaf) –
Gently grab the top with both hands and fold two-thirds down, then tug the left side across the middle and right side across the middle over the bit you just folded over. Finally, grab the bottom with both hands and pull over your folds. Turn it 90 degrees and roll into a sausage, then place into a banneton seam-side up.

Shaping a boule (round loaf)
Pull the sides of the dough into the middle, starting at the top and going all the way round until you get a tightened ball. Flip it and use the sides of your hands to spin it on the countertop tightening the skin. Then place in a banneton or bowl, seam-side up.

Step 7 – Leave to rest on the counter for up to 30 minutes – it should be nice and jiggly when you pop it into the fridge. Leave the loaf in the fridge uncovered for 10–24 hours before baking.

To bake, preheat a lidded pot (see equipment) in the oven for 30 minutes at 230°C fan/250°C/475°F/gas mark 9. Tip your loaf onto a piece of parchment, score and gently lift into your hot pot. Bake with the lid on for 45 minutes. Allow to cool completely (at least 1 hour) before slicing.

NOTES
Using a finely milled wholemeal flour will give you a light loaf and yet all the fibre. If you find the dough too sticky and hard to work with, try making it with all white flour a few times to practice. Once you have mastered the basics, you can increase the proportion of wholemeal flour. Flours tolerate different levels of hydration; usually wholemeal can manage more water. If you are increasing your proportion of wholemeal flour, also increase water up to 400g (14 oz).

GUT-FRIENDLY ADDITIONS

To boost your bread, you can make additions when you add the salt. If adding flax seeds or chia seeds note that they soak up quite a bit of water so you might want to add another 25g (1 oz) as you squish them in. Stick to about 50g (1¾ oz) flax or chia.

Sunflower, pumpkin, sesame or poppy seeds are all great additions, as well as chopped nuts and dried fruit. You can add up to 100g (3½ oz) at the same time as adding salt. Note that they will firm up your dough a little but can make it more difficult to handle, so it is best to play with additions once you've nailed the basics.

USEFUL EQUIPMENT

- **Mixing bowl**

- **Dough scraper**

- **Digital scales**

- **Banneton** (suitable for 1kg/2lb 4 oz) dough) or a bowl or colander covered with a tea towel, plus rice flour to dust.

- **Lame** (razor blade in a holder) or a very sharp knife or serrated knife to score.

- **Baking vessel** a Dutch oven is best, about 5 litre capacity but a lidded Pyrex, or lidded enamel or ceramic roaster can also be used. Check maximum temperature tolerance before baking and reduce oven temperature if needed.

TROUBLESHOOTING

My bread is gummy/flat/dense

The loaf could be underbaked, cut into too soon or, most common, under-proofed. This happens a lot to beginners, don't despair, make sure your starter is active and happily doubling and increase bulk proof next time.

My bread is flat as a pancake

A flat loaf will usually be due to either under-proofing or over-proofing the dough. Under-proofing is more common than over-proofing. Study your crumb, if dense and gummy, and maybe some large but irregular holes it is typically underproved. If webby and flat, it's most likely overproved. A well-fermented crumb will have a mixture of hole sizes, be quite 'lacey' in appearance and have no dense areas. If very sticky to handle when shaping, or 'floating out' when tipping out to bake, the dough could be under- or over-fermented (your crumb will tell you which). However, it could also be a lack of tension and strength in your dough. Work on doing enough stretch and folds during bulk, and better shaping. Shaping is hard at first, but practice makes perfect.

My dough won't rise

If you struggle to judge fermentation, it can be a good idea to prove in a square see-through plastic container, allowing you to mark the side so you can track rise. Slow or lacking rise is often due to the starter not being strong and active enough. Feeding it twice a day for a couple of days can help give it a boost, as well as using finger warm water both for feeding and mixing the dough. Be mindful of temperature – if your kitchen is cold, finding somewhere cosy to prove can help (like the middle rack of the oven, switched off, with a bowl of just-boiled water, or put the pilot light on for 15 minutes to warm it up a little).

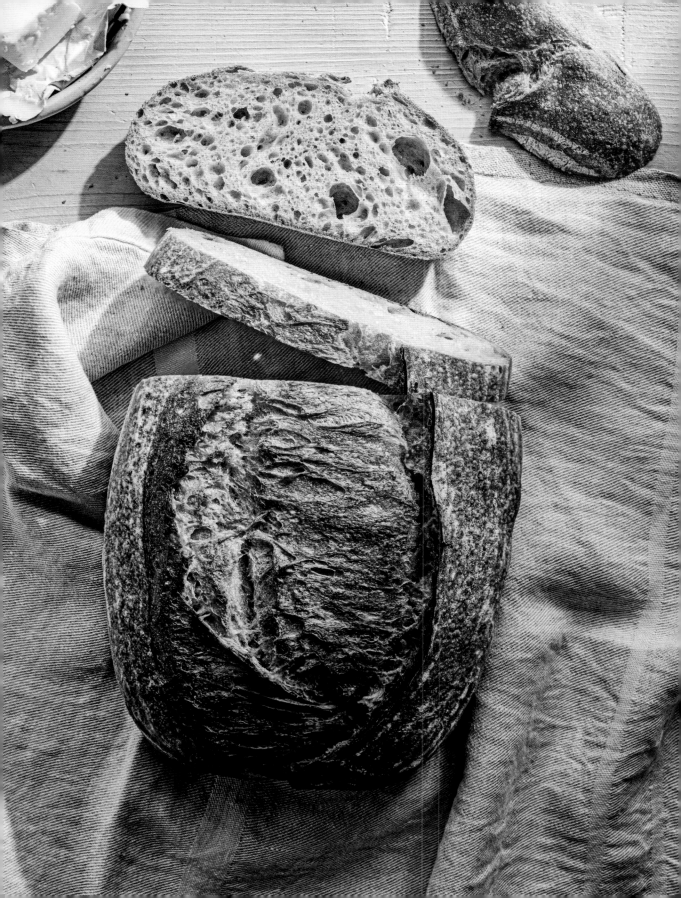

the gut stuff sauerkraut

Name: Sour cabbage (goes by 'sauerkraut').

Likes: Hummus, potatoes and toast.

Dislikes: Being left out on the side too long.

Describe yourself in a few words: I'm tangy, sweet-smelling and make any dish complete.

50 minutes prep | Serves 20 portions
+ 7–14 days fermenting

1 cabbage *(green or red)*
sea salt
1 tbsp fennel seeds
   (optional)

1. Wash a 1-litre (1¾-pint) jar in hot soapy water, then place it in the oven at 90°C fan/110°C/225°F/ gas mark ¼ for 15–20 minutes to sterilize it. Leave it to cool.

2. Remove the outer leaves of the cabbage and, if you're not using a weight, set a cabbage leaf aside. Slice into quarters and remove the hearts. Finely slice the quarters into thin ribbons.

3. Place a mixing bowl on a set of scales and zero the scales. Place the sliced cabbage into the mixing bowl and measure its weight. Calculate 2% of that weight (multiplying by 0.02) and measure out the result in

salt. Sprinkle the measured salt over the cabbage and add the fennel seeds, if using. Using your hands, begin to squeeze the cabbage and massage for 5–10 minutes. The salt will draw water out of the cabbage, creating its own brine. Leave the mixture to sit for 30 minutes.

4. Pack the cabbage into the sterilized jar, being sure to add in all the cabbage juices, then pack down the contents by compressing the reserved cabbage leaf over the top, or by using a weight. Ensure you're applying enough pressure so that the brine covers the shredded cabbage completely.

David Zilber is a chef, fermenter, food scientist and co-author of the NYT bestselling cookbook, The Noma Guide to Fermentation. He's basically the Rhianna of the fermenting world.

David Zilber: *If you start off making this sauerkraut recipe with white cabbage, you can easily liven it up and turn it into a carotene dream. You simply need 2 good nubs of turmeric root, 1 young carrot, and tiny sweet potato (or, roughly the same amount of sweet potato as carrot by weight). Peel the sweet potato (as its skin is fairly fibrous), but simply wash the carrot and turmeric, so you retain all of the potent nutrients that sit just below the surface. From there, brunoise or finely mince all three of the roots. Toss the glowing mix into the bowl with the shredded cabbage before you measure 2% of its weight in salt, but continue with the recipe as normal from that point on. Other, optional seasonings that would fare well in this recipe and sunny up any cloudy day include: a tablespoon of dill pollen, caraway seeds, or toasted yellow mustard seeds.*

5. Cover the jar with a burping lid and leave it at room temperature, out of direct sunlight. After 24 hours, press down the cabbage again using the weight or leaf to ensure that the cabbage is submerged beneath the brine.

6. Start to taste test after 7 days. Once the sauerkraut has reached your desired tanginess, replace the burping lid with a screw-top lid, cover securely.

Store in the fridge for up to 4 months. We like ours around day fourteen – it's just the perfect level of tang!

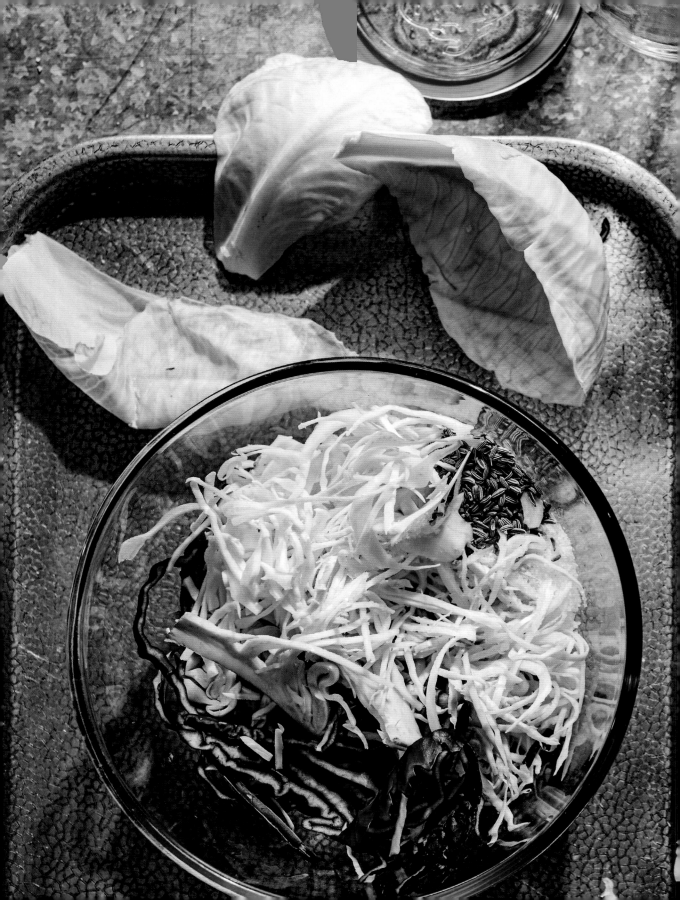

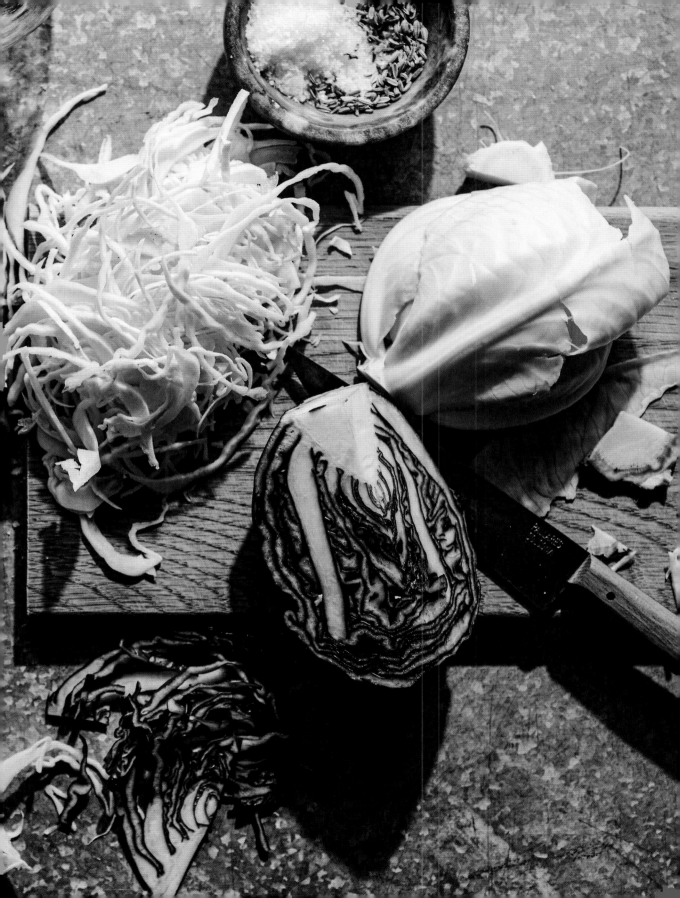

kimchi

Name: Kimchi

*Likes: Lactic acid, as many vegetables as possible, chilli, rice, cheese and buddha bowls...
what a versatile soul.*

Dislikes: Mould and being left unattended somewhere warm.

*Describe yourself in a few words: Spicy, sour and smelly enough to clear a crowd
(just what you're looking for from a date!).*

....

20 minutes prep | Serves 20
+ 12 hours resting
+ 7–14 days fermenting

1 Chinese leaf cabbage
(napa cabbage)

1 litre (1¾ pints) water

2 tbsp sea salt

2 carrots *(skin on)*

100g (3½ oz) radishes

bunch of spring onions

6 large garlic cloves

2 shallots

2 red chillies

100g (3½ oz) fresh ginger,
peeled

1–3 tbsp Korean chilli flakes
or cayenne pepper

2 tbsp tamari *(optional)*

....

1. Wash a 1 litre (1¾-pint) jar in hot soapy water,
then place it in the oven at 90°C fan/110°C/225°F/
gas mark ¼ for 15–20 minutes to sterilize it. Leave it
to cool.

2. Remove the outer leaves from the cabbage and
discard them, then rinse the rest of the cabbage
head well and cut into thick (5–6cm/2–2½-in) strips.

3. Using a jug, make a brine by mixing the water and
salt. Stir well to ensure the salt is well dissolved.
Place the sliced cabbage into a large bowl and pour

the brine over the leaves to cover. Cover the bowl
with clingfilm or a lid if it has one and leave it at
room temperature overnight.

4. The following day, drain the brined cabbage,
reserving the brine.

Recipe continued overleaf

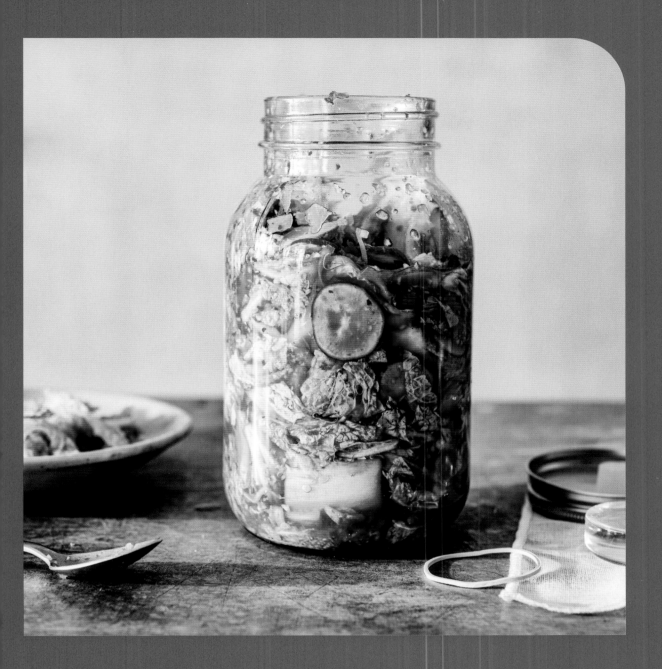

David Zilber: *While the above ingredients are considered near universal stalwarts of kimchi recipes around the world, kimchi can encompass so much more than cabbage (and can be considered an umbrella term for a style of pickling). To get at the 'roots' of that sentiment, try a kimchi with radishes as its star; 250g (9 oz) D'Avingnon radishes, 250g icicle radishes, 250g Shunkyo radishes and 250g mini mak (you can disregard the 100g/3½ oz radish the original recipe calls for, but keep everything else the same). Cut all the radishes into similar-sized quarters, lengthwise, and treat them as you would the cabbage in the original recipe. The finished product is a crunchily delectable variation that's enlivens any meal it's served with.*

5. Grate the carrots, chop the radishes into thin slices and roughly chop the spring onion. Peel the garlic and shallots, deseed the chillies.

6. In a blender (or using a knife to finely mince), make a paste with the ginger, garlic, deseeded red chillies, shallots and chilli flakes or cayenne pepper (depending on your desired spice level). Transfer the paste to a large mixing bowl with your brined cabbage leaves and add the grated carrots, sliced radishes, spring onions and tamari (if using). Using rubber gloves, massage the mixture into the vegetables for 5–10 minutes.

7. Pack the vegetables tightly into the sterilized jar and cover with a little reserved brine, if required, to ensure it sits beneath the level of the brine-line.

8. Place a weight on top to ensure that everything stays beneath the brine-line, and securely seal the jar with a burping lid.

9. Store your jar at room temperature for 7–14 days. Begin tasting your kimchi after 7 days. It should be salty, pleasantly sour and a bit crunchy with the flavours melding together harmoniously. When fermented to your liking, replace the burping lid with a screw top lid.

Store in the fridge for up to 4 months.

fermented garlic

Likes: Kissing.

Dislikes: The fact that nobody likes kissing me.

Describe yourself in a few words: Like a lava lamp, bubbly, mesmerising and hot ;)

This recipe could not be easier!

10 minutes prep | Serves 7
+ 5–7 days fermenting

allergens: *garlic*

2 heads of garlic
300ml (10 fl oz) room
    temperature water
½ tsp sea salt

1. Wash a 500ml (18-fl oz) jar in hot soapy water, then place it in the oven at 90°C fan/110°C/225°F/gas mark ¼ for 15–20 minutes to sterilize it. Leave it to cool.

2. Peel the garlic cloves and add them whole to the jar. Add the water to a jug with the salt and stir until it has dissolved. Cover the garlic with the brine. If the garlic is not submerged under the brine, add some baking paper to weigh it down. Add the burping lid and leave at room temperature for 5–7 days.

3. Begin tasting after 5 days. Once the ferment has reached your desired taste, replace the burping lid with a screw-top lid and move to the fridge.

Store in the fridge for up to 4 months.

milk kefir

―――

Name: Kefir (key-feh).

Likes: Lactose.

Dislikes: Getting too hot (ooo-er).

Describe yourself in a few words: I've been around for centuries – I'm creamy, tangy and contain more microbes per ml/fl oz than yogurt.

MILK KEFIR YOGURT

To make milk kefir yogurt, follow the recipe below. After removing the grains, re-seal the jar and store at room temperature for a further 12–24 hours to thicken. Once thickened, store in the fridge and use within 4 days.

....

2 minutes prep | Serves 20
+ 24–48 hours fermenting

5g (⅛ oz) milk kefir grains
250ml (9 fl oz) whole milk

allergens: *cow's milk*

....

1. Wash a 500ml (18-fl oz) jar in hot soapy water, then place it in the oven at 90°C fan/110°C/225°F/ gas mark ¼ for 15–20 minutes to sterilize it. Leave it to cool.

2. Add the milk kefir grains to the sterilized jar and pour the milk over the top. Gently stir with a clean spoon to evenly distribute the microbes. Cover with gauze and fix in place with a rubber band. Set aside at room temperature for 24 hours, away from direct sunlight.

3. After 24 hours, stir and judge its taste and consistency. When the milk has thickened and tastes pleasantly tangy, it's ready. If not, replace the gauze and rubber band and continue fermenting at room temperature for a further 24 hours.

4. Once ready, strain the jar's contents through a sieve over a bowl to catch the final kefir. Transfer the milk kefir to a clip-top bottle and cover tightly.

Store in the fridge for up to a week.

water kefir

Name: Water kefir (water key-feh).

Likes: Special grains, sugar and water.

Dislikes: Being abandoned or heated metal spoons and sieves.

Describe yourself in a few words: I'm hungry, a quick grower, effervescent, slightly fruity and definitely alive!

10 minutes prep | Serves 4
+ up to 4 days fermenting

20g (¾ oz) cane sugar
800ml (1½ pints) filtered water *(room temperature)*
30g (1 oz) water kefir grains

1. Wash a 1 litre (1¾-pint) jar in hot soapy water, then place it in the oven at 90°C fan/110°C/225°F/ gas mark ¼ for 15–20 minutes to sterilize it. Leave it to cool.

2. Add the sugar to the sterilized jar, followed by the water and stir until the sugar has completely dissolved. Then add the water kefir grains. Gently stir the liquid once more to distribute the microbes throughout, then cover the jar with gauze and secure it tightly with a rubber band. Set aside at room temperature for 48 hours, keeping the jar away from direct sunlight.

3. After 48 hours, strain the grains from the mixture using a sieve and reserve. Pour the brewed kefir water into a clip-top bottle, then either store in the fridge or leave it out for another 48 hours to carbonate further.

Store in the fridge for up to a month, unopened. Once opened, it is best consumed within 30 days.

kombucha

Name: Kombucha *(kom-boo-cha, replacing sam-boo-ka), or 'booch' for short.*

Likes: Fruity flavours and symbiotic cultures of bacteria and yeast.

Dislikes: Being left out too long and stainless steel.

Describe yourself in a few words: Fizzy, fruity and sometimes so tart I'll make you pucker up!

....

10 minutes prep | Serves 7
+ 1 hour cooling
+ 5–7 days fermenting

1.7 litres (3 pints) filtered water
120g (4¼ oz) cane sugar
4 black teabags
200ml (7 fl oz) finished kombucha from a previous batch (*or the liquid the SCOBY is packaged in*)
1 SCOBY

....

1. Wash a 2 litre (3½-pint) jar in hot soapy water, then place it in the oven at 90°C fan/110°C/225°F/gas mark ¼ for 15–20 minutes to sterilize it. Leave it to cool.

2. In a large saucepan, bring the water and sugar to the boil. Stir to dissolve the sugar, then remove the pan from the heat and add the teabags. Steep for 5–10 minutes. Remove the teabags and leave to cool to room temperature.

3. Add the mixture to the sterilized jar, followed by the finished kombucha and SCOBY and cover the jar with gauze, fixing it in place with a rubber band. Leave the jar at room temperature but out of direct sunlight.

4. Fermentation can take anywhere from 5–14 days, depending on your desired taste. Begin tasting the kombucha after five days. As the kombucha ferments, its sugary sweetness will diminish as its

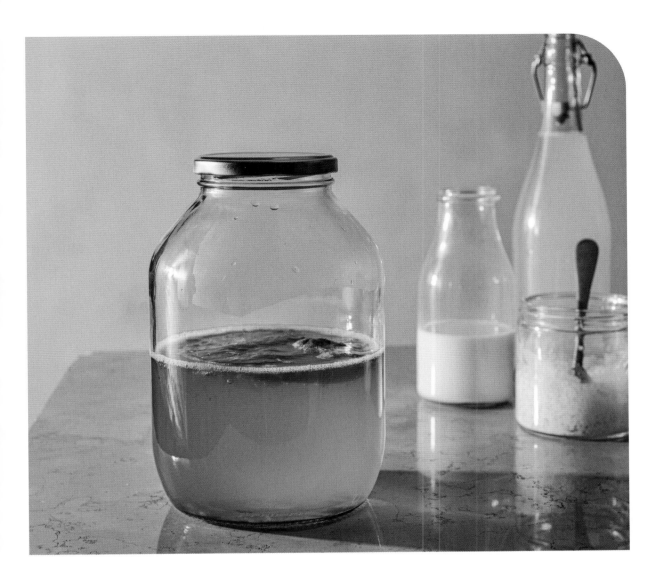

acidity rises. Once it has reached your desired level of tanginess, remove the SCOBY and reserve 200ml (7 fl oz) of kombucha to brew your next batch.

5. Strain the finished kombucha through a sieve to remove any stray particles that may have formed during fermentation. Use a funnel to pour your brewed kombucha into a clip-top bottle, then either store in the fridge or leave it out for a further 48 hours to carbonate further.

Store in the fridge for up to a month unopened. Once opened, it is best consumed within 7 days.

6. Repeat the process using the SCOBY and reserved kombucha to make a fresh batch of kombucha.

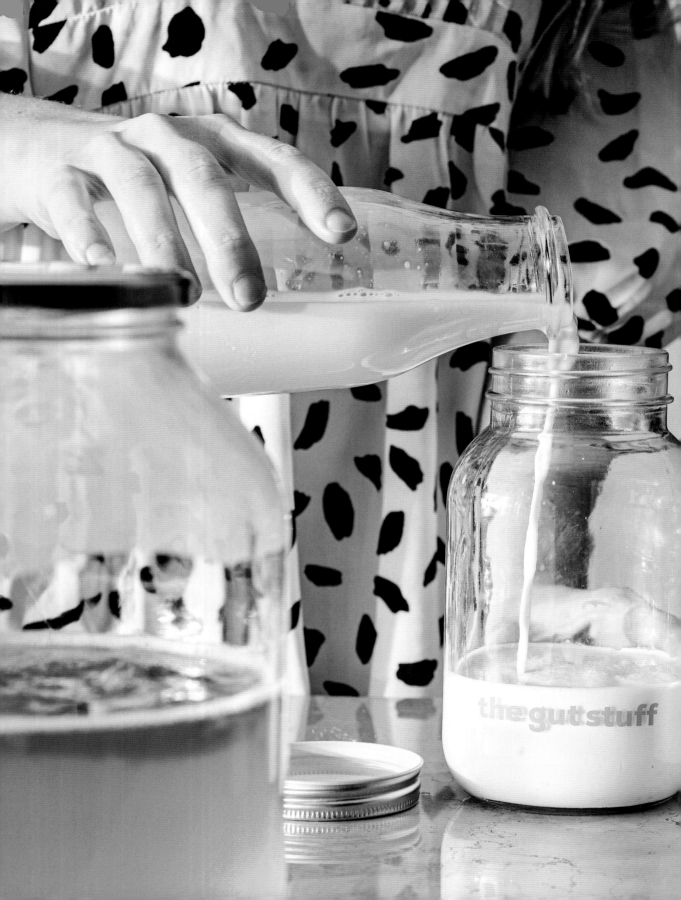

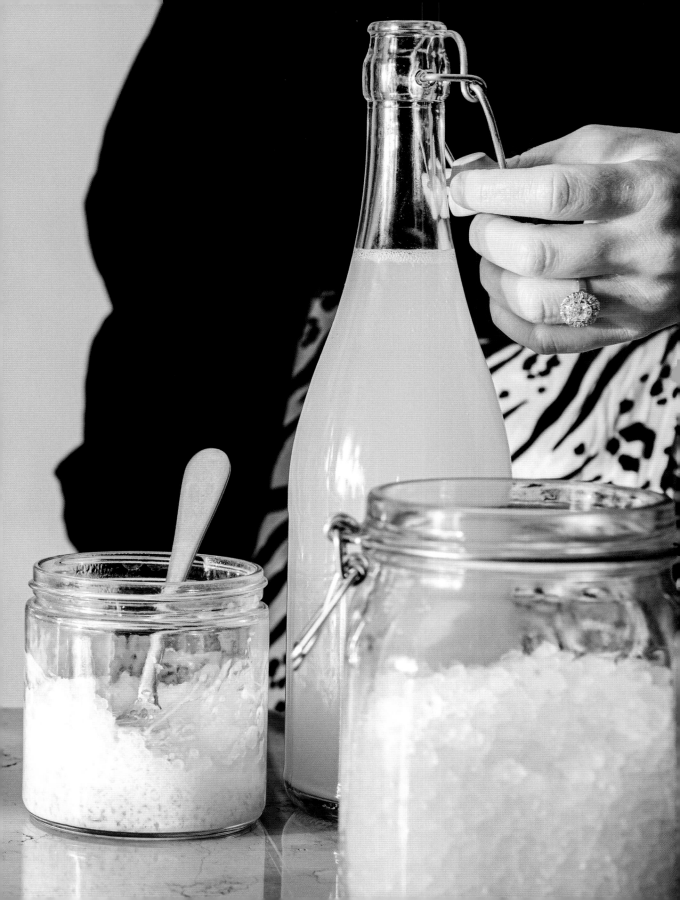

UK–US cooking terms

Aubergine – **eggplant**

Baking paper – **parchment paper**

Baking tray – **baking sheet**

Beetroot – **beet**

Black-eyed beans – **black-eyed peas**

Butter beans – **lima beans**

Cake tin – **cake pan**

Chestnut mushrooms – **cremini mushrooms**

Chickpeas – **garbanzo beans**

Clingfilm – **plastic wrap**

Coriander – **cilantro**

Courgettes – **zucchini**

Frying pan – **skillet**

Little Gem lettuce – **Boston lettuce**

Loaf tin – **loaf pan**

Pak choi – **bok choy**

Passata – **strained tomatoes**

Pepper (red, yellow, green) – **bell pepper**

Rocket – **arugula**

Tomato purée – **tomato paste**

Wholemeal – **whole wheat**

gut glossary

bacteria

what is it?
Bacteria are single-celled micro-organisms and can be found all over our bodies, including our mouths, skin and, of course, our gut.

There are so many different species of bacteria in your gut. Think of the different species as having different job titles – they all do different things.

Within a bacteria species (or job title), there are 'strains'. Strains are a further way of separating out the differences between bacteria belonging to the same species. For example:

Species: *Lactobacillus* (music artist)
Strains: *L. acidophilus* (bassist)
　　　　 L. amylovorus (DJ)
　　　　 L. casei (singer)
　　　　 L. rhamnosus (backing vocalist)

what does it do?
Mostly, lots of great things, but sometimes the wrong type or too many/too few bacteria can cause problems.

The bacteria in your gut make up your microbiota. The ratio of human to bacterial cells is thought to be 1.3:1. Scientists are continuing to research the true ratio, but it makes up a big proportion of who we are!

bile

what is it?
Bile is a liquid produced in your liver and stored in your gallbladder. Your gut microbes can influence your bile and bile can influence your gut microbiota.

what does it do?
Bile helps us break down fats so we can absorb fat-soluble vitamins, such as vitamins A, D, E and K. It also gets rid of toxins we no longer need.

chyme

what is it?
Chyme is a cocktail of stomach acid, digestive enzymes, partially digested food and water.

what does it do?
Chyme allows for further digestion by enzymes and is a carrier of food and enzymes to the small intestine.

dysbiosis

what is it?

Think of your gut microbiota as a country garden – you want a variety of different plants (beneficial microbes) and not too many weeds (less beneficial microbes) for a happy and healthy gut. We need our gut microbiota to be diverse and balanced to work at its best. If it is in a state of dysbiosis, this means it is imbalanced or there is a disturbance in the normal composition of microbes, for example, decreased diversity of beneficial microbes.

what does it do?

Dysbiosis may negatively affect different aspects of your health, including your immune system and physical and mental health.

enzyme

what is it?

Digestive enzymes are crucial for good gut health! Your body produces lots of different digestive enzymes to support the digestion and the absorption of fats, proteins, carbohydrates and micronutrients. For example, amylase is secreted by your salivary glands and pancreas to break carbohydrates down into glucose, which your body can use as fuel, and lipase is secreted by the pancreas to support fat digestion.

what does it do?

Digestive enzymes help to break down our food so we can absorb it. If we don't break down our food properly, it can affect our gut microbes.

faeces

what are they?

This is just another word for poo! Faeces are made up of water, bacteria, fats, proteins, toxins and undigested food, including fibre, which helps bulk out your stool.

what do they do?

The purpose of having a poo is to rid your body of waste, toxins and other compounds

fibre

what is it?

Fibre is a type of carbohydrate either naturally derived from plants or extracted and added into a product (isolated fibre). Unlike some carbohydrates, fibre cannot be digested in the small intestine and so passes through to the large intestine where the magic happens. It is an essential nutrient for your gut and your gut microbes to thrive.

There are many different types of fibre. You'll often here the term soluble and insoluble – this just refers to whether it can be dissolved or not in water. Splitting up fibre in this way doesn't really tell us much about the effect it has on the body and your gut will differ depending on the types of fibre and proportions found in any given food.

what does it do?

Fibre has many important uses in the body.

- Fibre bulks out and softens your stool by retaining water, which supports gut transit time and prevents constipation.
- Certain types of fibre can be fermented by beneficial gut bacteria, which produce short-chain fatty acids, which are a source of energy and also have other health benefits.
- Fibre slows the breakdown of sugars found in carbohydrates, which helps to stabilize your energy levels.
- Fibre promotes an environment favourable to beneficial gut bacteria.
- A diet high in fibre can reduce the risk of developing high cholesterol, heart disease, diabetes and bowel cancer.

gut-associated lymphoid tissue (GALT)

what is it?

Yes, it is a bit of a mouthful, but GALT is extremely important and a huge part of your immune system! It consists of lots of immune cells lining your gut and it plays a fundamental role in defending your body against foreign invaders.

what does it do?

Protects you from pathogens such as bacteria and viruses. Your gut microbiota can influence how well your GALT works and vice versa.

gut

what is it?

When we talk about the gut, we mean your small and large intestine. Your small intestine has an average length of 3–6 metres! Your large intestine (where the majority of your gut bugs live) is around 1.5 metres long and makes up one fifth of your digestive tract. Your large intestine houses most of your gut bacteria. Your gut is supported by your stomach, liver, pancreas and gallbladder.

what does it do?

Your gut has many functions, but the key ones are:

- houses the majority of your microbiome
- digests and absorbs nutrients
- supports immune function
- plays a role in producing chemicals that affect how we feel

In your lifetime, around 60 tonnes of food will pass through your gut!

gut microbiome

what is it?

The trillions of microbes, their functions and genes (including bacteria, yeast, fungi and parasites and their genetic material) living within your gut. More than 1,000 species have been identified!

what does it do?

Our microbiome does incredible things, here are our top pics:

- Produces vitamins, including vitamin K and B vitamins
- Produces short-chain fatty acids, which fuel your gut cells
- Supports immune function and defends against pathogens
- Influences how often you 'go' to the loo
- Regulates the health of your gut
- Ferments fibre that your body cannot digest
- Influences mood and mental health
- Influences sleep
- Supports hormone regulation
- Regulates metabolism

gut microbiota

what is it?

The types of organisms (bacteria, viruses, parasites etc.) present in your gut. You might also hear the terms 'microbiota' or 'microflora' used interchangeably, but we use the term microbiota.

Diet, medication, environment and genes are just some of the factors that can influence your gut microbiota.

Our microbiomes are unique to each and every one of us! Twins may have the same DNA, but their microbiomes will be different.

Our gut bugs can determine how well we manage different foods, from bananas to avocados.

what does it do?

Your microbiota is responsible for:

- Produces vitamins, including vitamin K and B vitamins
- Produces short-chain fatty acids, which fuel your gut cells
- Supports immune function and defends against pathogens
- Influences how often you 'go' to the loo
- Regulates the health of the gut
- Ferments fibre that your body cannot digest

Your microbiota is responsible for:

- Produces vitamins, including vitamin K and B vitamins
- Produces short-chain fatty acids, which fuel your gut cells
- Supports immune function and defends against pathogens
- Influences how often you 'go' to the loo
- Regulates the health of the gut
- Ferments fibre that your body cannot digest
- Influences mood and mental health
- Influences sleep
- Supports hormone regulation
- Regulates metabolism

Your gut microbes interact with almost all of your human cells!

gut mucosa

what is it?

The gut mucosa includes GALT (see page 273) as well as other immune cells and bacteria, which all work together to distinguish friend from foe in the gut. It allows dietary substances to cross into your bloodstream but still stops pathogens form entering. Specific types of bacteria like to live in your gut mucosa, like our old friend *Akkermansia*.

what does it do?
An important part of our immune system, which provides a balance of beneficial bacteria and stops pathogens from getting in.

polyphenols

what are they?
Polyphenols are protective compounds found in plants; typically they are found in higher quantities in brightly coloured vegetables. Your gut microbiota converts polyphenols from plants into something your body can use.

Food sources include brightly coloured vegetables, fruit, tea, coffee, chocolate (at least 75% cocoa solids), legumes and some cereals.

what do they do?
Polyphenols have antioxidant properties, support your microbes to be their best selves and support overall health.

prebiotics

what are they?
Prebiotics are a specific type of fibre, which can be broadly defined as non-digestible carbohydrates. Our gut bacteria like to ferment them, which can cause changes to our gut microbes.

The following are types of prebiotic fibre you might hear about:

• Inulin
• Oligofructose
• Galacto-oligosaccharides (GOS)
• Xylooligosaccharides (XOS)

Great sources of prebiotic food include onions, garlic, leeks, bananas, asparagus, artichokes, olives, plums and apples, plus wholegrains like oats and bran and nuts, such as almonds.

what do they do?
Prebiotic foods can change the composition of your gut microbes by stimulating growth of beneficial bacteria.

probiotics

what are they?
The term 'probiotic' is banded around a lot! The true meaning is a live micro-organism that, when administered in adequate amounts, confers a health benefit on the host. Probiotics can be in food or supplement form, but not all probiotics are created equal – different strains have different effects, and some might have no effect at all. It all depends on the individual. Examples of food probiotics include yogurt, kimchi, sauerkraut, kefir, miso and kombucha. BUT if you are buying shop-bought versions, make sure you check for 'live bacteria' on the back of the pack.

what do they do?

Depending on the strain and the individual, probiotics can have lots of positive effects on the person consuming them. Some examples of what they can do:

• compete with other microbes in your gut
• effect your gut mucosal barrier
• support your immune system

Science is still learning exactly how different strains work, so watch this space.

short-chain fatty acids

what are they?

Most short-chain fatty acids are produced within your large intestine following the fermentation of fibre by your gut microbes.

The main types are:
Acetate
Propionate
Butyrate

Each have different functions in the body. Fermented products may also contain short-chain fatty acids. If we don't eat enough fibre, this can decrease the amount of 'food' that bacteria have to ferment and therefore reduce the number of short-chain fatty acids produced.

what do they do?

Short-chain fatty acids keep your gut healthy, are the primary source of energy for gut cells, are involved in the metabolism of nutrients (including carbohydrates and fat), support your immune system and may be protective against certain diseases.

We are still learning about the role of short-chain fatty acids and health.

gut conditions

Candida

Candida is a type of fungus or yeast that grows all over the human body, especially in warm and moist areas like the mouth, stomach and vagina. The presence of candida isn't usually a problem unless an overgrowth occurs. Although overgrowth is quite common, the severity of these infections varies greatly. Candida overgrowth is also called: Candidiasis, a Candida infection, a yeast infection, a fungal infection and Thrush.

Clostridium difficile
(C. diff as it's known to its pals)

You may have heard of this bacterium. It can infect the bowel and cause diarrhoea (in healthy individuals it is unlikely to cause an issue because beneficial bacteria keep it in check). Symptoms include diarrhoea, high temperature or tender stomach.

Coeliac disease

Coeliac disease is an autoimmune condition whereby your body's own immune system attacks itself when gluten is eaten (even very small amounts like cross contamination). This causes damage to your small intestine and can result in malabsorption meaning you won't be able to absorb the nutrients from food. Your doctor is always your first port of call if you think you have Coeliac disease.

Crohn's disease

Crohn's disease is a type of inflammatory bowel disease. It can cause inflammation in any part of the gut but mostly occurs in the last section of the small intestine or large intestine. It is a chronic condition but periods of remission mean the individual can be symptom free at certain times. It can impair digestion and absorption of nutrients and how well your body gets rid of waste. Symptoms vary as different sections of the gut are affected. Main symptoms are diarrhoea, stomach aches/cramps, blood in your stools, tiredness and weight loss. Symptoms can be managed with medication and in some cases, surgery.

Diverticular disease and Diverticulitis

These are both conditions affecting your large intestine. As we age, small pockets appear in the lining of our large intestine – these are called diverticula. The presence of diverticula does not mean you will experience symptoms, but some people do. If you have no symptoms but have diverticula, it is called diverticulosis. If you have symptoms, such as stomach pain, it is called diverticular disease. Sometimes the diverticula can become infected or inflamed increasing the severity of symptoms – this is called diverticulitis.

Digestive cancers

Digestive cancers include:
Colorectal cancer, also known as bowel cancer, which develops in the large intestine or rectum. Gastric cancer, where cells form in the stomach lining. Pancreatic cancer where cells form in pancreatic cells. Other cancers considered rare affecting the digestive tract.

Dumping syndrome

Dumping syndrome is a term to describe a range of different symptoms occurring when food is too quickly evacuated from the stomach in to the small intestine, resulting in undigested food that hasn't been digested properly making it difficult to absorb nutrients. It has different causes and is common after bariatric surgery (also known as bypass surgery).

Gallstones

Most gallstones consist of cholesterol and are made in your gallbladder. They often go un-noticed but sometimes they can get trapped trying to get out, causing intense stomach pain.

Gastrointestinal malabsorption

Gastrointestinal malabsorption is where you are unable to fully absorb nutrients from your gut, which, if the underlying cause is not treated or managed, can cause malnutrition. The most common cause is Coeliac disease, Crohn's disease and pancreatitis. Symptoms include weight loss, impaired growth in children, chronic diarrhoea, fatty and greasy stools and fatigue.

Gastroparesis

Gastroparesis is a chronic condition causing the contents of the stomach to empty slower than it should. It is caused by an impairment in muscular and nerve communication. There are multiple reasons behind its cause, including complications with type 1 and 2 diabetes, Parkinson's disease, and complications from surgery, such as bariatric surgery and gastrectomy. Symptoms include feeling very full (quickly), nausea and vomiting, loss of appetite, weight loss, bloating and stomach discomfort and heartburn.

H. pylori

Helicobacter pylori is a type of bacterium. An *H. pylori* infection is a bacterial infection of the stomach, where the bacterium sets up home in the mucus layer of your stomach. It weakens the mucus and exposes the stomach lining; the bacteria then irritate the lining, resulting in an ulcer and inflammation. Some people may have an *H. pylori* infection but not experience symptoms. Common symptoms include abdominal pain, bloating, belching and nausea. It can be treated but requires medical attention.

Haemorrhoids (piles)

These are more common than you'd think. Haemorrhoids are swollen blood vessels and appear as lumps in or around your bottom. You are more likely to get them if you are constipated, strain too hard, during pregnancy and even heavy lifting. They can be painful and may result in bright red blood after you poo but always seek help from your doctor to rule out other causes.

Heartburn and reflux

Heartburn is a burning sensation in the chest caused by stomach acid or its contents being regurgitated and coming up into the oesophagus or throat (acid reflux). It commonly occurs after meals and when lying down. Up to 25% of UK adults are affected. Symptoms vary but include sore throat, heartburn, indigestion, bad taste and the sensation of a lump in your throat. If this occurs regularly, its proper name is gastro-oesophageal reflux disease (GORD). There are different underlying causes, including the sphincter at the bottom of your oesophagus/top of your stomach not working as well as it should.

Hernia

There are several different types of hernia. They occcur when an internal part of your body is pushed through muscle or tissue wall. The most common place is between the chest and hips. If you have a hernia, you will most likely notice a lump or swelling. Surgery may be recommended to treat it. If you think you have a hernia, please speak to your doctor.

IBS

Irritable bowel syndrome affects your digestive system. Symptoms include stomach cramps, diarrhoea, constipation, bloating, wind, mucus, nausea and tiredness – there are different types and your doctor will diagnose you. Symptoms can happen sporadically, last for days, weeks and even months. Scientists don't know exactly what causes IBS and it can be a difficult condition to live with. Symptoms can be managed but there is no cure. Keep a diary and speak to your doctor for further information.

Intestinal ischaemia

This is a rare circulatory condition and can affect your small or large intestine. It occurs where the arteries delivering blood to your gut are affected resulting in a reduced blood flow.

Oesophagitis

Oesophagitis is where the oesophagus (linking your stomach to your throat) becomes inflamed. This mostly occurs due to acid reflux. Not everyone with reflux will develop oesophagitis, it depends on the sensitivity of your oesophagus. Symptoms are similar to acid reflux, including pain in the chest and towards the neck, an acid taste in the mouth and pain swallowing hot drinks.

Pancreatitis

This occurs when your pancreas becomes inflamed either in a short space of time (acute pancreatitis) or over a long period of time becoming permanently damaged (chronic pancreatitis). Alcohol abuse is a common cause of chronic pancreatitis.

Short bowel syndrome

Short bowel syndrome happens due to physical loss or loss of function of a section of the small and/or large intestine. This may result in malabsorption of nutrients. Diarrhoea and malnutrition are common symptoms.

SIBO

SIBO stands for small intestinal bacterial overgrowth. This occurs when an unusually high amount of bacteria is found in the small intestine, which leads to uncomfortable symptoms in the gut. This can happen when there is an overgrowth of bacteria in the small intestine, or when bacteria moves from the large intestine into the small intestine.

Stomach/gastric/ duodenal ulcers

Stomach or gastric ulcers are ulcerations that occur on the stomach lining or first section of the small intestine. You may also hear the term peptic ulcer. It happens when the lining of the stomach breaks down causing damage. It can be caused by H.pylori infection or non-steroidal anti-inflammatory drugs like aspirin. Burning or abdominal pain are the main symptoms, but you may also experience indigestion, heartburn or nausea. Seek urgent medical help if you vomit blood, pass dark, sticky stools, have blood in your stools, sharp pain that gets worse.

Ulcerative colitis

Ulcerative colitis (UC) is a type of inflammatory bowel disease (you may hear it called IBD). It causes inflammation and ulceration of the large intestine and rectum (where stools are held before being released). The large intestine has a delicate lining and ulcers can form along it, which can cause bleeding and pus. Severity of symptoms will vary person to person but the main symptoms are diarrhoea (you may see blood, mucus or pus), stomach pain, frequent trips to the loo, fatigue, loss of appetite and weight loss and anaemia. Other symptoms are also associated with UC. It is an ongoing condition but symptoms can be managed with medication and, in some cases, surgery.

Seek help from your doctor if you are experiencing gut symptoms.

index

references

GUT SCIENCE
Louis, P. et al. (2009), "Diversity, metabolism and microbial ecology of butyrate-producing bacteria from the human large intestine", FEMS Microbiology Letters (294:1):1–8. DOI:10.1111/j.1574-6968.2009.01514.x

Zinöcker, M.K. et al. (2018), "The western diet-microbiome-host interaction and its role in metabolic disease", Nutrients, (10:3):365. DOI:10.3390/nu10030365

Carbohydrates and Health, Scientific Advisory Committee on Nutrition (TSO), 2015. ISBN:9780117082847

Myhrstad, M. et al. (2020), "Dietary fibre, gut microbiota, and metabolic regulation-current status in human randomized trials", Nutrients, (12:3):859. DOI:10.3390/nu12030859 2020

Sanders, M.E. et al. (2019), "Probiotics and prebiotics in intestinal health and disease: from biology to the clinic", Nat Rev Gastroenterol Hepatol, (16):605–616. DOI:10.1038/s41575-019-0173-3

Kumar Singh, A. et al. (2019), "Beneficial effects of dietary polyphenols on gut microbiota and strategies to improve delivery efficiency", Nutrients, (11:9) p2216, 2019. DOI:10.3390/nu11092216

The American Gut Consortium: McDonald, D. et al. (2018), "American Gut: an open platform for citizen science microbiome research", mSystems, (3:3):e00031-18. DOI:10.1128/mSystems.00031-18

Karl, J.P. et al. (2013), "Effects of psychological, environmental and physical stressors on the gut microbiota", Frontiers in microbiology, (9). DOI:10.3389/fmicb.2018.02013

Zheng, D. et al. (2020), "Interaction between microbiota and immunity in health and disease", Cell Res, (30):492–506. DOI:10.1038/s41422-020-0332-7

Martin, A.M. et al. (2019), "The influence of the gut microbiome on host metabolism through the regulation of gut hormone release", Frontiers in physiology, (10):428. DOI:10.3389/fphys.2019.00428

Rizzello, C.G. et al. (2019), "Sourdough fermented breads are more digestible than those started with baker's yeast alone: an in vivo challenge dissecting distinct gastrointestinal responses", Nutrients, (11:12):2954. DOI:10.3390/nu11122954

Koistinen, V.M. et al. (2018), "Metabolic profiling of sourdough fermented wheat and rye bread", Scientific reports, (8:1):5684. DOI:10.1038/s41598-018-24149-w

Reese, A.T. et al. (2020), "Influences of ingredients and bakers on the bacteria and fungi in sourdough starters and bread", mSphere, (5:1):e00950-19. DOI:10.1128/mSphere.00950-19

Melini, F. et al. (2019), "Health-promoting components in fermented foods: an up-to-date systematic review", Nutrients, (11:5):1189. DOI:10.3390/nu11051189

Bourrie, B.C. et al. (2016), "The microbiota and health promoting characteristics of the fermented beverage kefir", Frontiers in microbiology, (7):647. DOI:10.3389/fmicb.2016.00647

Lobionda, S. et al. (2019), "The role of gut microbiota in intestinal inflammation with respect to diet and extrinsic stressors", Microorganisms, (7:8):271. DOI:10.3390/microorganisms7080271

Davani-Davari, D. et al. (2019), "Prebiotics: definition, types, sources, mechanisms, and clinical applications", Foods (Basel, Switzerland), (8:3):92. DOI:10.3390/foods8030092

Carlson, J.L. et al. (2018), "Health effects and sources of prebiotic dietary fiber", Current Developments in Nutrition, (2:3):nzy005. DOI:10.1093/cdn/nzy005

Househam, A.M. et al. (2017), "The effects of stress and meditation on the immune system, human microbiota, and epigenetics", Advances in Mindbody Medicine, (31:4):10–25. PMID:29306937

Toribio-Mateas, M. (2018), "Harnessing the Power of Microbiome Assessment Tools as Part of Neuroprotective Nutrition and Lifestyle Medicine Intervention", Microorganisms, (6:2):35. DOI: 10.3390/microorganisms6020035

MENTAL HEALTH
Long-Smith, C. et al. (2020), "Microbiota-gut-brain axis: new therapeutic opportunities", Annu Rev Pharmacol Toxicol, (60):477–502. DOI:10.1146/annurev-pharmtox-010919-023628

Yang, B. et al. (2019), "Effects of regulating intestinal microbiota on anxiety symptoms: a systematic review", General Psychiatry, (32:2):e100056. DOI:10.1136/gpsych-2019-100056

KRISTY COLEMAN
Clark, A., Mach, N. (2016),

"Exercise-induced stress behavior, gut-microbiota-brain axis and diet: a systematic review for athletes", J Int Soc Sports Nutr, (13:43). DOI:10.1186/s12970-016-0155-6

Dalton, A. et al. (2019), "Exercise influence on the microbiome-gut-brain axis", Gut Microbes, (10:5):555–568. DOI:10.1080/19490976.2018.1562268

Das, M. et al. (2019), "Gut microbiota alterations associated with reduced bone mineral density in older adults", Rheumatology (Oxford, England), (58:12):2295–2304. DOI:10.1093/rheumatology/kez302

Mailing, L.J. et al. (2019), "Exercise and the gut microbiome: a review of the evidence, potential mechanisms, and implications for human health", Exerc Sport Sci Rev, (47:2):75–85. DOI:10.1249/JES.0000000000000183

JENNA MACCHIOCI
Tamburini, S. et al. (2016), "The microbiome in early life: implications for health outcomes", Nat Med, (22):713–722. DOI:10.1038/nm.4142

Salazar, N. et al. (2019), "Age-associated changes in gut microbiota and dietary components related with the immune system in adulthood and old age: a cross-sectional study", Nutrients, (11:8):1765. DOI:10.3390/nu11081765

Mowat, A.M. (2018), "To respond or not to respond – a personal perspective of intestinal tolerance"., Nat Rev Immunol,

correction (18:8) p536, original (18:6):405–415. DOI:10.1038/s41577-018-0002-x

The American Gut Consortium: McDonald, D. et al. (2018), "American Gut: an open platform for citizen science microbiome research", mSystems, (3:3):e00031-18. DOI:10.1128/mSystems.00031-18

Laitinen, K., Mokkala, K. (2019), "Overall dietary quality relates to gut microbiota diversity and abundance", Int. J. Mol. Sci, (20:8):1835. DOI:10.3390/ijms20081835

Rinninella, E. et al. (2019), "What is the healthy gut microbiota composition? A changing ecosystem across age, environment, diet, and diseases", Microorganisms, (7:1). DOI:10.3390/microorganisms7010014

Maslowski, K.M. (2011), "Diet, gut microbiota and immune responses", Nat Immunol, (12:1):5–9. DOI:10.1038/ni0111-5

Dimidi, E. et al. (2019), "Fermented foods: definitions and characteristics, impact on the gut microbiota and effects on gastrointestinal health and disease", Nutrients, (11:8):1806. DOI:10.3390/nu11081806

Mills, J.G. et al. (2019), "Relating urban biodiversity to human health with the 'holobiont' concept", Front. Microbiol, (10), DOI:10.3389/fmicb.2019.00550

Cox, L.M., Blaser, M.J. (2015), "Antibiotics in early life and obesity", Nat. Rev. Endocrinol,

(11:182). DOI:10.1038/nrendo.2014.210

SOPHIE MEDLIN
Patel, S.G., Ahnen, D.J (2018), "Colorectal cancer in the young", Curr Gastroenterol Rep, (20:4):15. DOI:10.1007/s11894-018-0618-9

Flynn, S., Eisenstein, S. (2019), "Inflammatory bowel disease presentation and diagnosis", Surg Clin North Am, (99:6):1051–1062. DOI:10.1016/j.suc.2019.08.001

Lacy, B.E., Patel, N.K. (2017), "Rome criteria and a diagnostic approach to irritable bowel syndrome", J Clin Med, (6:11):99. DOI:10.3390/jcm6110099

Lebwohl, B. et al. (2017), "Coeliac disease", Lancet. (391:10115):70–81. DOI:10.1016/S0140-6736(17)31796-8

Vijayvargiya, P., Camilleri, M. (2018), "Update on bile acid malabsorption: Finally ready for prime time?", Curr Gastroenterol Rep, (20:3):10. DOI:10.1007/s11894-018-0615-z

van der Heide, F. (2016), "Acquired causes of intestinal malabsorption", Best Pract Res Clin Gastroenterol, (30:2):213–224. DOI:10.1016/j.bpg.2016.03.001

Rezapour M. et al. (2018), "Diverticular disease: an update on pathogenesis and management", Gut Liver, (12:2):125–132. DOI:10.5009/gnl16552

CHRIS GEORGE
Pechey, R., Monsivais, P. (2016), "Socioeconomic

inequalities in the healthiness of food choices: Exploring the contributions of food expenditures", Preventive Medicine, (88):203–209. DOI:10.1016/j.ypmed.2016.04.012

WHO Health Topics, "Healthy Diet", World Health Organisation. URL:www.who.int/nutrition/topics/2_background/en/

WHO Global Health Observatory, "Noncommunicable diseases: Mortality", World Health Organisation. URL:www.who.int/gho/ncd/mortality_morbidity/en/

UEG, "Europe is 'failing' to deal with chronic digestive disease burden", United European Gastroenterology, 14 May 2018. URL:https://ueg.eu/a/43

LAURA TILT
Simren, M. et al. (2016), "Bowel Disorders", Gastroenterology, (150:6):1393–1407. DOI:10.1053/j.gastro.2016.02.031

McKenzie, Y.A. et al. (2016), "British Dietetic Association systematic review and evidence-based practice guidelines for the dietary management of irritable bowel syndrome in adults (2016 update)", Journal of Human Nutrition and Dietetics, (29:5):549–575 DOI:10.1111/jhn.12385

NICE (2008), "Irritable bowel syndrome in adults: diagnosis and management", NICE: Clinical guideline, (CG61). URL:www.nice.org.uk/guidance/cg61/

Drossman, D.A. et al. (2009), "International survey of patients with IBS: Symptom features and their severity, health status, treatments, and risk taking to achieve clinical benefit", Journal of Clinical Gastroenterology, (43:6):541–550. DOI:10.1097/MCG.0b013e318189a7f9

Drossman, D.A. (2016), "Functional gastrointestinal disorders: History, pathophysiology, clinical features, and Rome IV", Gastroenterology, (150:6):1262–1279. e2. DOI:10.1053/j.gastro.2016.02.032

SOCIAL EATING
Choi, K.W. et al. (2020), "An exposure-wide and Mendelian randomization approach to identifying modifiable factors for the prevention of depression", The American Journal of Psychology, (177:10):944–954. DOI:10.1176/appi.ajp.2020.19111158

Johnson, K.V.A. et al. (2022), "Sociability in a non-captive macaque population is associated with beneficial gut bacteria", Frontiers in Microbiology, (13). DOI:10.3389/fmicb.2022.1032495

Dill-McFarland, K.A. et al. (2019), "Close social relationships correlate with human gut microbiota composition", Scientific Reports, (9)703. DOI: 10.1038/s41598-018-37298-9

Johnson, K.V.A. (2020), "Gut microbiome composition and diversity are related to human personality traits", Human Microbiome Journal, (15):100069.

DOI: 10.1016/j.humic.2019.100069

Nguyen, T.T. et al. (2021), "Association of loneliness and wisdom with gut microbial diversity and composition: an exploratory study", Frontiers in Microbiolog, (12). DOI:10.3389/fpsyt.2021.648475

COVID
Natarajan, A. et al. (2022), "Gastrointestinal symptoms and fecal shedding of SARS-COV-2 RNA suggest prolonged gastrointestinal infection", Med, (3:6):371–387.e9. DOI:10.1016/j.medj.2022.04.001

Blackett, J.W. et al. (2021), "Prevalence and risk factors for gastrointestinal symptoms after recovery from Covid-19", Neurogastroenterol Motil, (34:3):e14251. DOI:10.1111/nmo.14251

Nakhli R.E. et al. (2022), "Gastrointestinal symptoms and the severity of Covid-19: Disorders of gut-brain interaction are an outcome", Neurogastroenterol Motil, (34:9):e14368. DOI:10.1111/nmo.14368

BIBLIOGRAPHY
Scott C. Anderson with John Cryan and Ted Dinan, The Psychobiotic Revolution: Mood, Food, and the New Science of the Gut-Brain Connection, (National Geographic, 2017)

Dr Jenna Macciochi, Immunity: The Science of Staying Well, (Harper Collins, 2020)

Anjali Mahto, The Skincare Bible: Your No-Nonsense Guide to Great Skin, (Penguin Life, 2018)

Renee McGregor, Fast Fuel: Food for Running Success, (Nourish Books, 2016)

Renee McGregor, Orthorexia: When Healthy Eating Goes Bad, (Nourish Books, 2017)

Renee McGregor, Training Food: Get the Fuel You Need to Achieve Your Goals Before During and After Exercise (Nourish Books, 2015)

Rosie Saunt and Helen West Is Butter a Carb? Unpicking Fact from Fiction in the World of Nutrition, (Piatkus, 2019)

Tim Spector, Spoon-Fed: Why almost everything we've been told about food is wrong, (Jonathan Cape, 2020)

Tim Spector, The Diet Myth: The Real Science Behind What We Eat, (Weidenfeld & Nicolson, 2016)

Kimberley Wilson, How to Build a Healthy Brain: Reduce Stress, Anxiety and Depression and Future-Proof Your Brain, (Yellow Kite, 2020)

WEBSITES & RESOURCES

Renee McGregor www.reneemcgregor.com

Sophie Medlin @sophiedietitian

Dr Rabia @doctor_rabia www.doctor-rabia.com

Ruari Robertson www.ruairirobertson.com

Laura Tilt @nutritilty

Laura Tilt @nutritilty

you've made it to the end!

From fibre and faeces to breathwork and brain health, what a journey this book has been.

We hope that not only have you got a grip on some of the science of your body (and around it!) but have also gained some tips on how to arrange your fridge, spot signs and symptoms and are even inspired to have go at fermenting. Once we all know why, it's so much easier to grasp the how and what as we have the impetus to make some positive changes, however small and incremental they may be.

We never expected this to be our path in life, but the importance and immediacy of finding out about and looking after our gut health has, quite literally, consumed us. We hope these pages have shown you even a fraction of our passion for this subject. We've brought together the all-stars from a variety of fields so you can see how widespread (and brilliant) this area of research is.

If you'd told us, aged 14, we would end up writing a book about gut health, we would have chucked our chips at you and shouted 'WITCHCRAFT!' But here we are. Life gets gutsier and more wonderful every day.

More than anything, we hope you feel empowered. Everyone has the right to know about their own bodies and, importantly, their guts, and be armed with the tools and confidence to make health and lifestyle decisions for themselves.

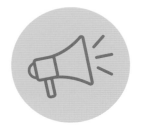

PS: Spread the good gut word and maybe pass this book on to a friend once you're done or visit our website **www.thegutstuff.com**

acknowledgements

Firstly, to our team at TGS HQ who have stuck by us on this business rollercoaster and everyday give us the incredible combination of heart and graft, we don't know where we'd be without you all.

To India who kicked this baby off with us, and everyone that believed in us from the very beginning, JKR and Revolt who sat in the tiny little sailboat with us as we set off on this journey... and the Haltons for giving us the strength when we thought we might sink.

To Shelly Nel who's warmth behind the camera was the catalyst for us to have access to the best scientists and professionals around.

To Luke and Peter, for the late nights and early mornings – thanks for standing by us.

To Mum who continues to hold our trembling hands when we step out of our comfort zone and to Uncle Brian and all the pals who read very early drafts and scribbles of these pages.

To our incredible community of followers – you are who we do this for.

And to everyone we've yet to empower – here's to the future.

To everyone who said to us all those years ago, what are you two on about?! Do you mean my beer belly? I hope now after reading this book you understand and share our passion to tell others. Onwards!

Lisa and Alana x